"A convincing and compelling testament to the value of mind-body approaches to healing and their integration into the mainstream of Western medical practice. Dr. Oz is showing us not only the direction and shape, but also a glimpse into the heart and soul of the medicine of the future."
—Jon Kabat-Zinn, Ph.D., Executive Director, Center for Mindfulness in Medicine, Health Care, and Society, University of Massachusetts Memorial Medical Center

"Dr. Oz provides interesting, informative descriptions and definitions of the alternative healing systems and provides insight into the relationships between the human nervous system and the control—even cure—of unusual human maladies. These complementary therapies represent a new direction in healing for mind and body alike."
—Denton Cooley, M.D., President and Surgeon-in-Chief, Texas Heart Institute

"Oz's case histories are fascinating, his skill and dedication undeniable, but what is most compelling here is the way he looks beyond the mechanics of his work to see each patient as a whole person."
—Yoga Journal

"An encouraging book in a field that always needs such close looks at itself."
—Booklist

Dr. Mehmet Oz, a highly respected cardiovascular surgeon, is the director of Columbia Presbyterian Medical Center's mechanical heart-pump program and is the cofounder and medical director of the hospital's breakthrough Complementary Care Center. As part of the innovative surgical team at Columbia Presbyterian, he also helped to develop the left ventricular assist device (LVAD), a high-tech artificial heart that keeps patients alive while waiting for a heart transplant. A dual U.S.-Turkish citizen from birth, Dr. Oz sees himself as a bridge between the healing ways of the West and the East. He lives with his family in the New York City area.
Ron Arias is a correspondent for *People* and the author of many books.
Lisa Oz is a writer, producer, actress, and mother.

Healing from ❧ the Heart ❧

*A Leading Surgeon Combines Eastern
and Western Traditions to Create
the Medicine of the Future*

Mehmet Oz, M.D.

with Ron Arias and Lisa Oz

FOREWORD BY DEAN ORNISH, M.D.

A PLUME BOOK

PLUME
Published by the Penguin Group
Penguin Putnam Inc., 375 Hudson Street, New York, New York 10014, U.S.A.
Penguin Books Ltd, 27 Wrights Lane, London W8 5TZ, England
Penguin Books Australia Ltd, Ringwood, Victoria, Australia
Penguin Books Canada Ltd, 10 Alcorn Avenue, Toronto, Ontario, Canada M4V 3B2
Penguin Books (N.Z.) Ltd, 182–190 Wairau Road, Auckland 10, New Zealand

Penguin Books Ltd, Registered Offices: Harmondsworth, Middlesex, England

Published by Plume, a member of Penguin Putnam Inc. Previously published in a Dutton edition.

First Plume Printing, October, 1999

10   9   8   7   6   5   4

Permission has been granted to reprint the extracts from the following books:

Rhodes, Peter. *Aim: The Workbook*. San Francisco: J. Appleseed and Co., 1994.
Wilson, Colin. "The Reality of the Visionary World," from *Testimony to the Invisible: Essays on Swedenborg*. James F. Lawrence, ed. Westchester, PA: Chrysalis Books, 1995.

Ⓟ   REGISTERED TRADEMARK—MARCA REGISTRADA

The Library of Congress has cataloged the Dutton edition as follows:

Oz, Mehmet.
    Healing from the heart: a leading surgeon combines eastern and western traditions to create the medicine of the future / by Mehmet Oz, with Ron Arias and Lisa Oz; foreword by Dean Ornish.
      p.   cm.
    Includes bibliographical references (p. 185).
    ISBN 0-525-94410-9
        0-452-27955-0 (pbk.)
    1. Alternative medicine.   2. Heart—Diseases—Alternative treatment.
I. Arias, Ron.   II. Oz, Lisa.   III. Title.
R733.095   1998
616.1'206—dc21   98-4573
                                                                  CIP

Printed in the United States of America
Set in Goudy
Designed by Eve L. Kirch

To teachers in all their forms:
our parents, colleagues, patients, and children

CONTENTS

AUTHOR'S NOTE

While all the case stories in this book are factual, in some cases the names of the patients have been changed to protect their privacy.

FOREWORD

Mehmet Oz is a physician for the new millennium: one who integrates the best of Western allopathic medicine— drugs and surgery—with an explorer's willingness to examine alternative approaches to health and healing that is both open-minded yet discriminating.

Dr. Oz is a first-rate cardiovascular surgeon, the epitome of high-tech Western medical intervention. He helped develop methods for implanting in people the left ventricular assist device, a complex, partial artificial heart to help keep patients alive while waiting for a heart transplant. He is technically proficient, but he is more than just a technician.

The heart is a pump and needs to be addressed on a physical level. However, our hearts are more than just pumps, and a true physician is more than just a plumber or a mechanic. We also have an emotional heart, a psychological heart, a spiritual heart.

Our language reflects that understanding. We yearn for our sweethearts, not our sweetpumps. Poets and musicians and artists and writers and mystics throughout the ages have described those who have an open heart or a closed heart; a warm heart or a cold heart; a compassionate heart or an uncaring heart. Love heals. I think these are more than just figures of speech.

Healing may occur even when curing is not possible. Curing when the physical disease gets better. Healing is a process of becoming whole.

When the emotional and spiritual heart begins to open, the physical heart often follows. For the past twenty years my colleagues and I have conducted a series of scientific studies demonstrating that the progression of even severe coronary heart disease often can begin to reverse by making comprehensive changes in diet and lifestyle. Since this had never before been shown, these approaches were considered by most physicians to be unconventional, alternative, even radical when I began doing this research. Now these ideas have become much more mainstream because we have been able to document the scientific validity and efficacy of these approaches.

Like Dr. Oz, I believe in the value of science in helping to sort out what works from what doesn't work, for whom, and under what circumstances. The fact that there is much in the alternative medicine world that is unproven does not mean that it is not worth examining. The true scientist—like Dr. Oz—retains the dual qualities of both open-mindedness and skepticism. As he asserts, only with hard, convincing data can a fundamental change in how we practice medicine come about.

In *Healing from the Heart*, Dr. Oz shares with us his voyage of discovery and what he has learned from his patients: how to harness the mind and body as an ally in healing the heart on all levels. His patients showed him their different worlds, revealing something deeper than their physical symptoms, scars, and lesions.

In their own language and stories, Dr. Oz describes how his patients began opening their hearts to him, allowing him to gain a greater understanding of how their emotions, attitude, and spirit affected both the physical aspects of heart disease and their experience of it. In turn, he began opening his heart to them and through his book—to us. As both Dr. Oz and his patients helped each other to become more whole, they became healers for each other.

Gradually, he began offering his patients more than just his surgical skills and medical knowledge. When undergoing surgery, patients give up all control during the operation. Vegetarian diet, guided imagery, massage, therapeutic touch, relaxation techniques, music, aromatherapy, and other unconventional modalities helped relax many of them, reducing their perception of pain after surgery and hastening recovery. More important, they helped these patients regain a greater sense of control by becoming more actively involved in their healing.

As Dr. Oz describes, he and his patients embarked on a life quest together. This book is a tale of that journey. It does not purport to be a definitive examination of complementary medicine or alternative healing. Rather, it is the story of how a respected mainstream physician, a dynamic surgeon at the leading edge of medical technology, came to explore the use of integrative medicine with his patients.

He asks: Why can't we be more tolerant of the unfamiliar? Why don't we adopt a more open, inquisitive view of healing? After strictly testing these therapies, why don't more hospitals offer effective integrative-medicine approaches to complement the more conventional treatments that are based on drugs and surgery?

Now more than ever, the medical profession needs physicians and scientists who have the courage and curiosity to bridge both worlds. For the question is not whether or not people should be using alternative-medicine approaches—they already are. In 1993 a widely reported article by Dr. David Eisenberg of Harvard Medical School reported that more money is spent out of pocket for alternative medicine than for conventional medicine. Unfortunately, many of these treatments are unproven and unstudied; some may be effective, others may be worthless or even harmful. We need more research to find out.

In the meantime, Dr. Oz provides compelling evidence from his own experience of the value of many of these approaches to him and his patients. *Healing from the Heart* gives us a glimpse into what the future of medicine is likely to be—if we're lucky.

> —*Dean Ornish, M.D.*
> *Clinical Professor of Medicine*
> *School of Medicine, University of California,*
>   *San Francisco*
> *President and Director*
> *Preventive Medicine Research Institute*

Hearken to this Reed forlorn
Breathing, even since 'twas torn
From its rushy bed, a strain
Of impassioned love and pain.

"The secret of my song, though near,
None can see and none can hear.
Oh, for a friend to know the sign
And mingle all his soul with mine!

'Tis the flame of Love that fired me,
'Tis the wine of Love inspired me.
Wouldst thou learn how lovers bleed,
Hearken, hearken to the Reed!"
   —The Song of the Reed
    by Rumi Mevlana, poet and mystic,
    of Konya, my father's hometown

A surgeon must have the eyes of an eagle,
the heart of a lion,
the hands of a woman,
the gentleness of a lamb,
the patience of a saint,
and the bladder of an elephant.
  —from medical lore,
   as modified by Dr. Bashir Zikria,
   Professor of Surgery, Columbia University

PROLOGUE

Cutting Edge

The heart has its reasons
that the reason knows nothing of.

—Blaise Pascal

I took a deep breath, looked down at the man's chest, and called out, "Ten blade!" A surgical nurse slapped the handle of the knife onto my right palm. With my left hand feeling for the middle of the chest bone, I raised the blade and with one swift motion cut the skin along an imaginary line from just below the patient's chin to his navel. The skin split apart like a neat zipper, as whitish fat tissue pushed to the surface and tiny rivulets of blood began filling the seam.

I had made this same cut in countless other surgeries, always with a mixture of excitement and trancelike focus. But this time the pressure on me and the surgical team to succeed had been raised a few notches. I was about to transplant a donor heart into a sixty-four-year-old man whose name had hit the headlines, and expectations for us to save his life were high.

As I cauterized the bleeding capillaries, I imagined Frank Torre, the anesthetized man now beneath my hands, as the hero of the 1957 World Series between the Milwaukee Braves and the New York Yankees. Just before Torre hit his first home run in the

series, he must have focused on the pitcher's fastball with all the
intensity of a cat about to pounce on its prey. He swung and
smacked the ball over the right-field fence, helping his team win
the game and later the championship. Now his brother Joe,
manager of the Yankees, faced a similar challenge in trying to
coach his team to one more win and a second World Series
championship in the Torre family.

I finished closing the last tiny bleeder, then called for the
electric saw, which was plugged in and handed over to me by its
metallic handle. "Drop the lungs," I ordered, and the anesthesiologist temporarily stopped the lungs from breathing. I asked for
power, and the saw's motor revved up to a dentist-drill's whine.
Covered by latex gloves and thin blue masks, caps and gowns,
the surgical team members watched as I pierced the upper notch
of the breastbone and carefully guided the blade toward the abdomen. I asked for more power, and the saw cut through the
bone like soft pine. My colleague Eric Rose and I both pulled on
the divided bone, and the chest parted. The heart, usually twisting and squeezing like a freshly caught fish in a bucket, lay slug-
gish and pumping feebly in the open chest cavity.

Frank Torre would die without a healthy donor heart, but as
his surgeon I was confident about the chances of a successful
transplant. I had spent most of my adult life learning how to
evaluate and treat patients like Frank. Four years at Harvard
College, four years at the University of Pennsylvania Medical
School, then seven tough years of surgical training, both general
and cardiac, at Columbia-Presbyterian Medical Center. All this
effort had thoroughly prepared me for thousands of subtle moves
my hands would have to make to replace Frank's sick heart with
a healthy one.

Fortunately, Frank was also thoroughly prepared. He had
trained hard for the transplant ordeal, which batters the patient's
mind as well as his body, with expert coaching to fortify the
single-minded determination that had made him a winner as a
baseball player. He was being treated with state-of-the-art high-

tech machinery, the most sophisticated, high-wire surgical techniques, plus another dimension of medical treatment that is just as cutting-edge, "complementary care." Complementary therapies include such ancient approaches to illness and well-being as simple yoga stretches, meditation, music, aromatherapy, and therapeutic touch—or "energy" healing, in which the healer's hands float inches over the body, never touching the skin. Combining these alternative therapies with the more familiar Western or "allopathic" approaches—surgery and drugs—was as revolutionary in American medicine as the groundbreaking heart transplants we were performing.

I first heard of Frank Torre's plight one morning in the summer of 1996. The initial call came from his family. Frank Torre's younger brother, Joe, who had lost a third brother to a heart attack only months before, was determined to keep his remaining brother alive. Frank himself didn't really want to know about his condition. He was afraid of what doctors would tell him, afraid the verdict would be a death sentence, that we would say he was beyond our help. Eventually Frank's brother and sister convinced him to come to Columbia-Presbyterian's cardiac unit for treatment and possibly a transplant.

We rushed him by ambulance from the airport. Once he was admitted, we immediately started giving him intravenous medications, followed by various diagnostic tests. Later, while talking to him, I could see the fear and apprehension in his eyes. I recognized that, aside from any surgery I would perform, my job would be to get him to change his attitude, from one of denial and fear about his illness to a positive approach for regaining a healthy life.

"So can you fix me?" Frank asked.

"Mr. Torre," I said, "we can help you if we work together."

One problem heart-transplant patients face is an often maddeningly unpredictable waiting period for donor hearts. Patients may remain in the hospital for months and sometimes more than a year, hooked up to life-saving equipment or dependent on drugs and constant monitoring, never knowing when they'll be summoned to take the fateful trip to the OR. The wait, the helplessness, and the hospital setting all conspire to make patients feel hopeless, anxious, and depressed. As I explained the ordeal ahead to Frank, I emphasized that to prepare himself for the transplant, he would have to take charge of some aspects of his care. Just as he had learned to play the game of baseball, he would now have to learn the "game" of medicine, to help himself get well.

From the start, Frank appeared to be open to an attitude change. Though he had retired decades ago as a player, the former first baseman was still strong and burly. We discussed the Yankees' fortunes that season and their winning spirit, which I pointed out could be a parallel to his own winning attitude toward his heart problem.

"That's going to be *my* attitude when I do the transplant," I said. "We're all on the same team, and you can't be a spectator. You have to be a player."

I referred Frank to Jery Whitworth, co-director of the hospital's Complementary Care Center. Besides being an operation-room perfusionist—the person who runs the heart-lung bypass machine during open-heart surgeries—Jery is also a trained hypnotherapist. In their first consultation, Jery found Frank a little skeptical of what many patients interpret as the "touchy-feely" school of medicine. An enthusiastic veteran at briefing new patients on some of these treatments, Jery started with the least New Age–sounding treatment, explaining that a proper hypnotherapy session—not some Las Vegas club act—might actually help him feel better physically and mentally while he and his clogged-up heart awaited the transplant. Before and after the surgery, hypnosis and other relaxation techniques might even reduce Frank's need for pain medication—important because such drugs can depress heart function or cause patients to lose touch with reality.

"What's the downside?" Frank asked at one point.

The downside? A waste of time, at worst, if Frank proved to be a poor candidate for hypnosis. Hypnotherapy treatments would do him no harm. As a former professional athlete, Frank knew the value of being calm and concentrated before each game, and so he could imagine the benefits of hypnosis. So Jery ran a quick test to see how susceptible Frank was to hypnotic suggestion.

"Close your eyes and extend both arms straight ahead," Jery said. "Now imagine your right arm is as light as a balloon. It's as light as air. It wants to float upward, higher and higher, just like a balloon, up into the air."

Jery told Frank to think of his left arm as a heavy piece of metal, thick and solid, very heavy, like lead. "You can barely lift it," Jery said. "It's so heavy, so very heavy."

When Frank was told to open his eyes, he was surprised to see his right arm raised a foot or so higher in the air than his left arm.

Frank's ready response to Jery's suggestions showed that hypnosis might prove a powerful aid for him before, during, and after surgery. Just as his conscious mind had interpreted the idea that one arm was a balloon and the other a piece of metal and his subconscious mind had levitated one arm and lowered the other, Frank would lower his heart rate, stabilize blood pressure, calm his breathing to a normal level, and relax his muscles until he felt like overcooked spaghetti.

Although he was a good candidate for hypnotherapy, Frank took to another therapy, reflexology, as if it were the ultimate elixir for good health. A therapy with roots in ancient Egypt, Greece, and China, reflexology is designed, so say its practitioners, to correct or relieve "imbalances" in the body that may be causing illness by manipulating different pressure points on the feet—toes, soles, sides, and heels—that correspond to different organs and parts of the body. Frank used to like what he called "that footsie thing" so much that his eyeballs would sometimes roll back and he would fall into a deep, restful sleep after a forty-five- to sixty-minute treatment.

Frank had to wait three months for a compatible donor heart to become available—time that he devoted to readying himself physically and emotionally for the surgery. As he was being wheeled into the OR, surrounded by the usual array of monitors, intravenous bags and tubes, he wore his game face—serious but serene.

"How're you feeling?" I asked.

"I'm ready," Frank announced in a matter-of-fact voice. I couldn't help thinking he'd been just as focused when he hit that home run in the '57 World Series.

I had given Frank a set of professionally developed tapes to listen to in his Walkman during surgery. The tapes featured soothing, gentle music with an overlay of spoken, repeated words: "Relax your neck, relax your shoulders . . ."—gentle commands repeated over and over like mantras to penetrate the unconscious mind and to reduce anxiety, relax muscles and lower the need for pain medications.

"So how are the tapes working?" I asked him.

Frank glanced up at me and shook his head slightly. "I can't listen to all that New Age stuff," he said. "It makes me feel like I'm going to a funeral. Just give me a little Nat King Cole." But the tapes helped. As I've noticed with many other heart-surgery patients using complementary medicine, Frank Torre showed little of the muscle tension and anxiety that other, more passive patients often show, and he had no big swings in blood pressure.

Inevitably, patients differ in what combination of complementary therapies they choose. Some, like Frank, take to one or two. Others go for everything, perhaps thinking that more is better or just to try them all before settling on what suits them best. Since every choice is voluntary, some patients completely reject such therapies, relying on prayer or their own fortitude. The saddest patients are those who seem to have given up the fight for life, who have retreated into a shell of silence and depression, and do not try anything at all.

Frank's positive spirit seems to have affected his brother's team during their improbable World Series showdown with the 1995 champion Atlanta Braves. While Frank was waiting for a heart that season, players and fans alike rooted for him as much as they did for the team. Then only hours after a 1–0 victory in Game 5, with the Yankees needing only one more game to win the championship, a matchable heart became available and Frank was next in line. Now the headlines shouted to win the game for Frank.

Under the powerful lights of the OR, while Frank was peacefully asleep with his Walkman on, I delicately lifted the donor heart from its blue and white Igloo cooler. Gently I place the organ in the center of Frank's vacant chest cavity, stitched it in, and then allowed the blood back into the heart. Within ten seconds the heart had changed from a limp brown lump marbled with patches of hard yellowish-white fat to a bright red, pulsing muscle. I poked it with a finger, and it twisted. I poked it again, and it stopped. Then I poked it a third time, and it sprang to life, quickly settling into the natural cardiac rhythm that has sustained Frank and all the rest of us since our lives began.

When Frank regained consciousness hours after the operation, I dropped by to check on his progress. "So how do you feel?" I asked him.

Still weak, groggy, and attached to various monitors and plastic tubes, he grinned and gave me a thumbs-up. "Like I played my own World Series," he said. "Pitched a no-hitter."

The next day, the Yankees beat the Braves. Frank's winning karma colored the city's celebration, right up to the ticker-tape parade a few days later.

Transplanting a heart is the culmination of everything I do as a surgeon. Particularly satisfying is the moment when life is reborn. The heart, after all, is the main engine and timekeeper of human life—what the sun is to the earth, a source of life-giving warmth and a regulator of days and nights, the heart is to the body. It nourishes our tissues with blood and sets our rhythm with a pulse. It is the physical wellspring of life.

And, some say, the wellspring of the soul. The heart is regarded as the center of human emotions. From the heart come fear, courage, love and hate. A heart can be light or heavy, aching or happy, crooked or pure. There are big hearts, open hearts, brave hearts, wild hearts, mighty hearts, bleeding hearts, and of course, broken hearts. In 1678 William Harvey, the famed English physician, wrote that the heart "is a household divinity which nourishes, cherishes and quickens the whole body, and is the foundation of life, the source of all action."

Since I was a child, the heart was *the* vital organ that riveted my interest, both in a physical sense and as an image. My fascination eventually led me on an exhilarating medical journey filled with discoveries—not just about what makes us tick but also about how we can enlist the mind to heal the heart.

The recovery of patients who have had open-heart surgery is often hindered by their perception that they have been abandoned by their hearts, their source of life, leaving them feeling emotionally and physically vulnerable. Drugs and modern medical technology may help keep these patients physically intact and functioning, but often they remain psychologically bereft with grief and a sense of worthlessness.

For this reason I soon came to recognize that responsibility could not end with the last skin suture I sewed. At the completion of the operation, no matter how successful, as a healer I also had to show the patient the path to recovery—a task made easier with complementary medicine treatments, particularly those that engage the mind to relax and lower fear, anxiety, and tension. These therapies can enable patients to pursue healing on their own—Frank Torre, for example, still continues his reflexology sessions several years after his transplant—and to grow through their illnesses, changing their perceptions about disease and healing.

My patients' stories of struggles, setbacks, and triumphs hold meaning for us all. Whether patients are beset by angina or asthma, the revolutionary comingling of conventional medical science and age-old remedies, of West and East, offers more complete and often more humane treatment than either healing approach by itself. My patients proved this to me, setting me on my own journey toward a more encompassing view of medicine, one that never underestimates the mind's role in healing the heart.

❧ 1 ❧

The Biology
of an MI

Any sufficiently advanced technology is indistinguishable from magic.
—Arthur C. Clarke, *The Lost Worlds of 2001*

What happens when a heart fails?

The heart is kept alive by three major arteries, or tubes, carrying blood to the heart tissue. Since the high-performance heart muscle is very sensitive to blood starvation, if these arteries close, the parts of the heart muscle fed by these vessels will die. If enough of the heart dies, not enough muscle will be left to keep pushing blood to the patient's brain and other vital organs, and the patient will die. Even if only a small part of the muscle dies, the dead tissue irritates the rest, causing irregular heart rhythms, which can also threaten life.

Let's look inside a coronary artery after an actual massive myocardial infarction (MI), which is the medical name for a heart attack. Let's call our patient Richard, a fifty-year-old accountant who has a blockage in one of his heart's three major arteries. What we see on the inside wall of the vessel are whitish fatty deposits, or plaque, which narrow the passage through which blood flows. Plaques usually consist of cholesterol, endothelial cells, and other scar-forming cells called fibroblasts. They can grow slowly and even form in young patients, as autopsies of soldiers killed in the Korean War demonstrated. Plaques tend to be hard and brittle, but sometimes on top of the rock pile of cholesterol-laden plaque we find a softer, granular sludge that is equally capable of stemming blood flow to the heart.

But a heart attack doesn't just happen because our vessels clog up like sewer pipes. Sometimes the chest pain results from the tendency of coronary arteries in some patients to spasm more than in others. While healthy vessels normally dilate during stressful times, diseased vessels are rigid. If Richard, for example, had a blockage of fifty percent but his blood vessels refused to dilate—because of chronic stress or a previously high-fat diet that caused hidden disease inside their walls—he would develop pain with minimal exertion or even in his sleep. But another person—let's say, an elderly woman whose heart disease is mostly hereditary—might have the same degree of blockage and no symptoms at all. Her heart disease might go undiscovered until she died of some unrelated cause—say, a car accident—and an autopsy revealed the blockage. So the physiological makeup of troubled arteries is an important factor in evaluating heart disease. How pliable, how spasm-prone are a patient's vessel walls?

Nor do "lesions," or narrowing of the coronaries, occur only in the spots where the most "gunk" or plaque has accumulated. They often occur at other, unexpected sites for reasons we don't yet know. In fact, a study of coronary-artery disease in sixty-two patients at St. Michael's Medical Center in Newark, New Jersey, shows that blockages may occur as commonly in relatively unclogged areas as in diseased arteries that are initially very narrowed.

Sometimes the buildup of plaque is slow enough that a complete blockage never occurs, or occurs after other open blood vessels "collateralize," or start to deliver additional blood to the area at risk. In such cases the MI is relatively mild. If Richard had built up another "collateral" blood system, he could have had a ninety-nine percent blockage without any symptoms and still be happily alive. Unfortunately, Richard had only a *fifty percent* blockage, and when it suddenly closed up, his heart had not had time to develop collateral vessels. Like many unsuspecting future MI victims, Richard—though his artery was only half blocked—paradoxically ran a greater risk for a big attack than some people with ninety-nine percent blockages.

Why would a fifty percent blockage suddenly close? The answer lies in what's in Richard's blood flowing past this lesser blockage, and also in the plaque's reaction to this blood. The surface of the plaque is very active and tends to be irritable. If a lot of blood elements, including sticky platelets, adhere to this surface, a fifty to sixty percent lesion can suddenly grow in size and close off all passage of blood. The plaque, like a balloon, can also fill itself with blood, expand, and plug the vessel.

What got Richard into this predicament? Nicotine might have led to hypertension. Too much cholesterol and dietary fat might have accelerated the chronic narrowing of his arteries. Maybe Richard, a guy with a button-popping gut, couldn't cope well with stress, which can lead to stickier platelets, hypertension, and dire results. He may have had a bad temper. When his patience finally popped in a snail-paced checkout line or his stored-up anger exploded in a highway traffic jam, the shoestring-size artery that was most vulnerable would have instantly squeezed down in a ripple of tightening spasms.

Studies show the most common time for an MI to occur is Monday morning, when the average middle-aged victim is back facing the firing line of work. Saturday morning ranks second, which may seem puzzling, since Saturdays are supposed to be more restful than working days. Yet if you have nothing to do, no errands to run, no hobbies or passions to pursue, the mere absence of activity can make you overly anxious. Another common time for MIs is during the early morning hours, when the body is asleep and working to digest fat-rich food eaten the night before. Platelets get stickier, and a vivid dream or just the stress of waking up can cause a clot to form, leading to a complete blockage.

When this happens, Richard feels a crushing, viselike pressure in his chest, pain shoots down his left arm, and he can hardly breathe as he dials 911 for emergency help. By the time he reaches the hospital, precious minutes have been lost while the affected part of his heart muscle is dying. Immediately after the ER doctor makes a diagnosis, Richard receives a potent blood thinner to dislodge the clot. When this fails, a dye is injected into his heart arteries through a catheter inserted into the groin's large femoral artery. A moving X-ray image on film—an angiogram—is then made of Richard's heart in full, crippled action, showing one major and several smaller blockages. The first-line doctors decide against angioplasty, a technique in which a tiny balloon near the end of a catheter is placed into the blocked artery and inflated, flattening the clot and the plaque and opening the vessel. Now Richard's only hope is open-heart surgery.

That's when I meet Richard. If I'd had the chance to get to know him before surgery, I could have introduced him to some of the complementary-medicine techniques we now use to relax patients, to help them become more confident and focused—in the zone or flow state, as I like to think of it. These techniques are especially helpful during some of the frightening and painful preoperative procedures that we must do without general anesthesia to avoid further reducing the patient's already poor heart function. For example, one of the first things we do in the OR is to stick a big needle into the patient's jugular vein, then snake a large-bore catheter down into the heart to measure certain chamber pressures. People who have undergone prior complementary therapies are often able to get through such procedures with less pain and anxiety than those who have not been trained to relax their throats, necks, and jaws.

But Richard's condition is so critical that we must operate immediately. He's just another draped and prepped patient waiting to have his chest opened, a name on a reel of angiogram film

I studied only moments before. All I can do to help him is to offer encouragement and try to talk him through the tough preoperative steps until we're ready to put him to sleep.

By the time I make the first deep incision in his chest, Richard has been in a deep sleep for about twenty minutes. It will take me almost an hour to connect the perfusion machine's plastic tubes to his aorta and the right atrium of his heart. Then, like a submarine captain shouting, "Down scope!" and "Dive!" I give the order: "Bypass on!" Jimmy, our perfusionist, manning the controls of the heart-lung machine, repeats, "Bypass on!" according to protocol. As I pinch off the aorta with a pliers-like clamp, I warn him: "Cross-clamp on, plegia up." Again Jimmy repeats the order and then begins infusing the preservative solution into Richard's heart. Bright red blood rushes through the pump's tubes into Richard's body, bypassing the heart and returning to the machine as a darker, oxygen-drained liquid. For the next fifty minutes Richard's bloodless, motionless heart remains still.

I snip a hole in his clogged, purplish coronary artery, which I will replace with a length of vein taken from his leg or with part of a mammary artery from under his upper ribs. First I meticulously pluck out several tiny loose bits of his blockage to prevent them from flowing downstream and blocking tributaries feeding the heart muscle. Then I sew the waiting vein to the diseased artery using polypropylene filament, the same material used in fishing lines but only a hair's thickness in diameter. My head loupes magnify the vein, the artery, and the tiny stitches I'm making by 3.5 times, enlarging my tiny working area to the size of a silver dollar. It's like a brightly lit miniature theater stage, and I've memorized the actors' faces and lines and motions perfectly.

The surgeon assisting me is positioned on the other side of Richard's body, and he also has both hands in the chest cavity. Together our twenty fingers do the precisely timed dance of snipping, holding, suturing, sponging, and swabbing that we've performed thousands of times since medical school. Then it's time to remove the cross-clamp so the blood can gush into Richard's newly attached vein, now serving as an artery, and flow back into the heart.

We wait a moment. The still motionless organ suddenly twists as the muscle contracts. A few seconds later it beats, then stops. Usually after a few false starts the heart will give a few tentative beats in a row, then flop like a fish, quickly assuming a reassuringly normal, regular rhythm as its pacemaker cells kick in. But in Richard's case the heart does not restart.

It's too late. Too much of Richard's very sensitive heart muscle is already dead. He needs a new heart, though the likelihood of finding one soon is very small, given the current critical shortage of donor hearts.

Fortunately, Richard's MI occurs at the end of the twentieth century, when we can save lives with a reliable mechanical pump like the Left Ventricular Assist Device (LVAD). So I implant an LVAD in him, which keeps his blood flowing until he gets a new heart months later.

If not for the LVAD, I might never have discovered the value of a formal program of such treatments as yoga, massage, hypnosis, therapeutic touch, and taped subliminal messages. The LVAD we use is a 2.5-pound titanium machine, about the size and shape of a portable CD player, which is implanted under the skin near the stomach to pump oxygen-rich blood out to the body, a process that is normally done by the heart's left ventricle. Powered by an external, hip-hugging battery pack, the metal gray device was developed by a group of Massachusetts engineers and scientists in the eighties so we could keep seriously sick and otherwise doomed heart patients alive while they waited for heart transplants.

To understand how this ingenious portable pump works, imagine that you are a blood cell. Every day your bone marrow makes millions of blood cells. Red ones carry oxygen to your body's tissues, after which they get recycled through your heart and lungs, then back again to your tissues. The red cells do this for about one hundred eighty days, then they die. The white blood cells roam around looking for intruders, like bacteria and viruses, to attack and kill. There are also platelets in your blood, sticky plugs that often take on amorphous shapes and are re-formed every seven days.

Imagine that you've just been created in bone marrow. But instead of being limited to being a red cell, white cell, or platelet, you belong to an elite cadre of cells, unique and gifted, because you have the power to become any cell you desire. Un-like most other tissues that have already differentiated—or cho-sen their purpose in life—you are still a free agent, able to play any role. You're called a "pluripotential-stem" cell. Most of your life is spent bathed in blood in the marrow. But every once in a while you may slip away into freely circulating blood and travel through the body. You careen through microscopic capillary beds; then suddenly you're ejected into a large vein—the inferior vena cava—that empties into the right side of the heart.

The muscles of this chamber contract violently, thrusting you into the lungs, where you meander through a bed of tiny alveoli. You are surrounded by a lining, a single-cell-layer in thickness that resembles onion skin. As your host breathes in and out, oxygen diffuses across this onion-skin barrier, while car-bon dioxide springs from the much more plentiful red blood cells all around you. Within seconds you're dumped into the most powerful blood muscle in the body, the left ventricle. Then wham! The chamber contracts. You rocket through the aorta and out to the rest of the body.

Now let's pretend that you are born in the bone marrow of an overweight fifty-year-old male whose father died of a heart at-tack in his fifties and who loves Camel cigarettes with strong Turkish tobacco. This man is having a fight with his wife as he reaches for another slice of pepperoni pizza. Suddenly he grabs his chest in pain and passes out, pink froth oozing down the side of his mouth.

Meanwhile you have just passed from his vena cava into the right side of the heart and are smashed into a backlog of cells that cannot get through the lungs. As your host's heart attack advances, the left ventricle can no longer contract strongly, and the blood backs up into the lungs, leaking through that onion-skin layer. Meanwhile the blood in the right heart chamber, or ventricle, can go nowhere and wells up in the liver and kidney, preventing those organs from working.

The patient, for now he has become one, is rushed to an emergency room. He's barely kept alive as we, the Left Ventricular Assist Device team, are called. ER physicians and nurses work frantically to reestablish a blood pressure and get a breathing tube down the airway passage. While they're trying to save him, we prepare the operating room for the inevitable. The patient is dying because not enough blood is reaching a big patch of his heart muscle. He needs an LVAD. And this we provide, opening his chest and abdomen to implant the fist-size pump and connect it to his heart.

You and the other pluripotential cells feel the difference immediately. The stagnant blood in the right ventricle gushes free into the lungs, then loops back to the left ventricle. But something is strange. This normally vigorous, forceful part of the heart is mute and lifeless, its chamber oddly still. Instead, you are sucked into a titanium tube, through a pig valve, and into a titanium chamber. Here you swirl around and around until you're ejected through another pig valve, up a cloth tube, and into the major vessel leaving the heart—the ascending aorta.

The next time through the circuit you notice that many of the other pluripotenial cells have stuck to the surface of the titanium pumping chamber and that this foreign body is looking remarkably like the rest of the host. An eddy in the current of blood sweeps you closer, pushing you into the lining. You stick on contact, but you feel comfortable. Rather than shriveling up, you expand tentacles and get a better grip. You and the other cells like you can finally stop your ravenous trips around the

body. You now densely pack yourselves together, content to pro-
liferate in your new, nutrient-rich home.

Before 1986 this would have been a made-up story. At the
time most heart surgeons viewed mechanical support as a failure.
Bud Frazier at the Texas Heart Institute in Houston was experi-
menting with a promising pump developed by Thermo Cardio-
Systems. Unlike the completely artificial Jarvik-7 heart that had
limited success in 1982 after it was implanted in several patients,
including Barney Clark, this new type of left ventricular assist
device worked in concert with a patient's existing heart in a
piggyback configuration. But even after many years of painstaking, trial-and-error research, the LVAD was not yet compatible
with the human body. Scientists and engineers had not been
able to solve a critical problem—preventing clots from forming
on the LVAD's inner surfaces, clots that would break away, lodge
in the brain, and cause strokes.

Then a unique set of developments convinced scientists that
instead of overpowering Mother Nature, they could fool the
body. How? They had always believed that a smooth surface
would be slippery enough to prevent small particles of clot from
forming and subsequently embolizing to various parts of the body,
causing strokes, among other complications. But these theories
failed in the ultimate mechanical-biological model—the human
body. Invariably, small defects in the lining or eddy currents
would promote clot formations, with resulting complications.

So what if the opposite approach—using a rough surface—
was taken? Blood would stick to a rough surface, but with the
right kind, it would adhere so smoothly that the cells could not
escape. When we tried this idea, our patients indeed had lower
stroke rates. But still no one knew why the theory worked, and
in order for any team to figure it out, it would have to have
access to large numbers of patients with LVADs. The crowded
New York metropolitan area was the perfect place to be.

In 1993, Eric Rose, my division chairman, recruited me to

build a Columbia Presbyterian LVAD program. During my surgical residency he had been my mentor, challenging me with difficult surgeries, then teaching me how to do the LVAD operation. So in the spring of 1994 I contacted the best basic scientists that I knew to work on the clotting problem. The group included experts in a range of fields, from cellular biology to bio-engineering. They were young—all under forty—eager researchers who had a high tolerance for heavy workloads. I still remember the critical meeting I called at three-thirty one morning in the operating room. I had just removed an LVAD from a patient prior to doing the heart-transplant surgery. I quickly carried the device over to a stainless steel tabletop, set it down in a pan, and opened both halves as if it were a clam. The team members gathered around to watch me take a scalpel and for the first time carefully slip the blade across the inside surface of the pump, slicing off a very thin layer of cells. I could sense the tension in the hands and arms of the young hematologist next to me as I dropped the cells onto the medium in the petri dish he was holding. He scurried off to the lab, knowing the little cells might hold the secret for saving lives. Over the next week the precious cells were nurtured and grown, then stained with specific markers to make possible their characterization.

By the time I reconvened the lab group for our weekly review and pestered them with questions about the lab results, we already knew we had made a major contribution to the field. Within a year we published our data on the pluripotential-stem cell and its unique ability to adhere to the titanium-sintered surface. For perhaps the first time bone-marrow cells had been observed growing in a patient outside the marrow. By encouraging them to grow in a thin layer inside the pump, we had finally hit on a way to mimic the amazingly clot-resistant lining of arteries. It was these talented cells that would eventually mature to the kind of cells that would populate the devices and make them safe.

The LVAD operates by taking in blood that flows through a tube grafted onto the apex, or tip, of the heart. The device pushes the blood out to the aorta and the rest of the body. At the same time the mechanically unassisted right ventricle takes care of pushing the blood through the lungs. So the blood goes from the heart into the device, circles around and back up to the aorta. The heart muscle itself contracts but doesn't do the left side's normal heavy work, which is to power oxygenated blood through the arteries and veins and back to the heart's right side. The left side stays limp, its big lower chamber, or ventricle, at rest. As I would soon discover, sometimes resting diseased hearts gained back enough strength so that when the LVAD was taken out, a transplant became unnecessary.

Eric Rose started implanting the devices, and at the same time began teaching me the procedure, but as division chief and then department chairman, he didn't have the time to build a strong mechanical-heart program. So I was in the right place at the right time. And with Eric's support I helped build one of the biggest and most active LVAD programs in the world. From 1993 to 1995 the number of LVAD patients waiting for new hearts at the hospital seldom dropped below six and sometimes rose to more than fifteen. Columbia-Presbyterian even started teaching surgeons at other hospitals how to implant the devices. Media coverage of our work also spread the word that we could offer not only the usual array of heart surgeries, but also several years' experience implanting LVADs, which, increasingly, were becoming the backup solution of choice if all other fixes failed. In time a prominent LVAD manufacturer even asked me if I could be available when Russian president Boris Yeltsin underwent bypass surgery. If it turned out that he needed an LVAD as a bridge to a transplant, I had agreed to do it.

The first devices were cumbersome, pneumatic-powered contraptions that patients had to push ahead of them like wheeled walkers. The suitcase-size machine contained a noisy compressed-air pump to power a piston-like plate propelling blood through the LVAD's chamber and out to the aorta. After more redesigning and clinical trials, the system matured. With every change we had to ensure that the theories of engineering meshed safely in the human body in which the pump had to function.

One young cardiologist, Dr. Howard Levin, who was also an engineer, knew the inner working of the device about as well as the manufacturer did. When devices started making abnormal noises or drawing excess amounts of electricity—harbingers of an impending malfunction—Howard had to develop algorithms for trouble-shooting the acute failures and new machines to diagnose more chronic abnormalities. Beat after beat, 60 times a minute, 3,600 times an hour, 86,400 times every 24 hours, 604,800 times a week—the pump had to work flawlessly.

LVAD hookups became one of the most fulfilling operations I did, in part because in each case it's not a question of *would* the patient have died without our help. He or she would definitely have died. In fact, by federal Food and Drug Administration requirements, before someone gets an LVAD, that person must clearly be near death. Treating LVAD patients was also fulfilling for other, non-surgical reasons. Because they required such close, continual attention, I saw a lot of the non-technical, emotional dimensions of healing, the kind best witnessed firsthand, not in a textbook or research paper. Patients felt abandoned, overwhelmed, scared, ambivalent, disgusted, angry, and/or confused. Was this my job to address? I was trained to diagnose and treat heart disease. Where did psychiatry and spirituality fit into my paradigm for treating patients? Wouldn't a few words of encouragement suffice?

I treated many of these patients almost daily for sometimes more than a year while they waited for their new donor hearts. I got to know them as few doctors get to know their patients, and such closeness helped precipitate a radical change in how I thought about health, disease, and illness. Ironically, it was allopathic medicine and the complexities of the modern hospital that would enable me to try older, simpler ways of healing my patients.

I remember, for instance, doing late rounds of the cardiac-patient floor one evening. I had just entered the central monitoring area when I spotted a cluster of bathrobed LVAD patients and a few of their spouses gathered in the lounge area they call the solarium, because of its large-window view of the Hudson River and the steep cliffs of the Jersey Palisades.

I was used to seeing my machine-tethered patients in the solarium, and on this night I spotted Betty D. and two of the men at a table under a single, hanging light. They were playing gin rummy and chatting with the bunch around them, which included a few nurses. Maybe because it was late and things were quiet everywhere else on the seventh floor, the scene looked out of place: lots of laughing, a baseball game blinking from the TV in the corner, people on vinyl-covered, cushioned chairs, snacks and soda pop cans on the end tables, and a half dozen of the old-style, air-driven LVAD walkers parked next to their users.

I paused by a bank of monitors and watched from a distance. The scene reminded me of similarly intimate gatherings I had attended during my childhood visits to Istanbul. On weekend evenings my parents and I would join the rest of the family at an aunt's house. The center of attention was a penny-poker game, played in the middle of a room under a single light. My father, two of my uncles, and a friend would sit around a table, and the rest of us who weren't in the game—kids, wives, friends—would sit right next to them in an outer circle. I'd wander among my relatives, now and then feeling an arm around my shoulders or a hand tickling my ribs. Mostly I was just happy to be woven into their lives.

Now, as I watched the friendly scene in the solarium, I knew these people were connecting in the same way. They knew each other's likes, dislikes, sleeping habits, the dates they had their LVADs implanted, how many months to the day they'd been waiting for their transplant, how many children each had, their names, even the names of their pets. Not many secrets were kept—they were comfortable confiding in each other. Unlike my more common bypass-surgery patients, who usually zip through post-op recovery in five or six days, these patients were pioneers in a new technology still being tested. Early LVAD patients had to live in the hospital, their bodies and devices monitored round-the-clock for problems. They weren't allowed home until they got donor hearts that their bodies were unlikely to reject.

I left the monitoring area and walked over to the card sharks and their audience. I didn't want to disturb the mood, but I also wanted to encourage them, keep their spirits high, even if only briefly.

"Hey Doc," one of the guys playing said, "Betty's winning again. What do you put in her IV drip?"

"I think she's winning on her own," I said with a wink in Betty's direction. "You're lucky you guys don't play for money."

We shared a strong feeling with LVAD patients that we were all in this together. When the program first began, the core team was composed of three people deeply committed to its success: Dr. Howard Levin, Kathy Catanese, a nurse, and Michael Gardocki, a physician's assistant. As soon as I finished implanting the device in a patient, this trio of professionals would take over. We all knew that the operation was only half the battle in prolonging life and that the team's role in successfully *managing* the patient's recovery was the other half. Howard oversaw the condition of the device and the patient's heart; Kathy, as the LVAD coordinator, took care of all the protocols and hospital logistics; and Michael helped by monitoring each patient's daily condition. Nutrition, physical therapy, medications, various tests—all had to be seen to twenty-four hours a day.

The newer generation of LVADs ejects ten liters of blood per minute. Warm, salty liquid filled with plastic-dissolving enzymes whooshes through the non-corrosive titanium chamber with metronomic efficiency, slowing down or speeding up as body needs dictate to built-in sensors. Rechargeable 1.5 pound battery packs provide the power, drugs decrease infections, and the fortuitous mimicry of pluripotential cells keeps killer clots from forming. Eventually, as the device became more portable and less cumbersome, patients could be discharged to live at home, only coming into the hospital periodically for checkups. The age of the artificial heart had arrived, thanks to the efforts of cracker-jack personnel.

Yet despite an appearance of normality in the lives of many LVAD patients, the goal of a transplant could never be forgotten. Wherever they went—and it couldn't be more than several hours away from our hospital—patients carried a pager and a cell phone. If a possible donor heart became available, the patient would be called to come in immediately for blood-matching tests and pre-op preparations. This is when the organ-harvest and transplant teams—composed of crack cardiologists, surgeons, physician's assistants and specialized nurses—entered the picture. I would perform the actual surgery, but these teams, starting with the LVAD trio of specialists, were the ones who brought the process to the point of surgery. Without them, the LVAD program could never have saved or prolonged so many lives.

By early 1994, with the LVAD program in full swing, I began to explore how my patients could benefit from a boost to their emotional lives. Card games and social intimacy were wonderful antidotes for loneliness and depression, but there were also many other ways to get people to heal, perhaps by harnessing their minds to the task. Death shadows LVAD patients more than most. They go into the operation, not for a transplant and an improved quality of life, but for a temporary solution, a quick fix dependent on a clever pump. Just the thought that they're artificially kept alive haunts some patients to a nearly neurotic state of fear and gloom.

At the home of Ivan Kronenfeld, I often reflected on my frustration with the inability of high-tech, successful interventions like LVADs to uniformly restore health at the home. An actor, writer, and an extremely religious man, Ivan was well read on the capabilities of the mind. At the small dinner table in his

Greenwich Village apartment, I would provide Ivan with the raw material of my cases. He would ferret out the bits of truth that would help guide him, me, and my patients toward a better understanding of how to restore health.

"What was your goal when you put in the LVAD?" Ivan would ask.

"To keep them alive," I'd answer. "Their hearts were dying."

"But why?" he persisted.

"So they would be able to breathe again, walk again, eat again."

"But has restoring their hearts restored their health?"

One of his favorite sayings is from the great physician and philosopher Maimonides: "The purpose of the study of wisdom is none other than its knowledge alone; and the purpose of truth is none other than to know that it is truth; and the purpose of knowing it is to do it."

Ivan was right. The LVAD was only the first step—albeit an essential, critical one. "The LVAD only gets them up," he would say. "You need to do *whatever is in your power* to make them healthy. That's what makes a healer."

About this time my wife Lisa gave birth to our youngest daughter, Zoe. In the hospital's maternity recovery room a torn piece of pink paper, crudely taped to the wall, advertised a massage service. This did not appear to be a hospital service, but at Lisa's urging I went ahead and made the call to someone named Rochelle.

When I returned later in the day, my wife looked rested and rejuvenated.

"What happened?" I asked.

"Rochelle came and gave me a massage," Lisa said. "I feel normal again."

I had purchased an inexpensive therapy that had had a major effect in improving my wife's well-being. Could my LVAD patients also benefit? I called Rochelle Aruti, introduced myself, and asked her how she was allowed to work in a hospital.

"Many years ago," Rochelle explained, "they grandfathered-in massage therapy for the maternity floor. It was controversial, but they allowed it."

"Can you do massage for my patients?" I asked.

"If you get me in, no problem."

A great idea had been sparked. The ability to bring even one massage therapist into the hospital would provide me with a foothold from which I could launch a formal program for offering complementary healing therapies.

I had begun researching how scientists study the nebulous concept of quality of life. I even applied for the prestigious Florence and Herbert Irving scholarship at Columbia University for funds to support this study. And I won. Now not only could I dedicate three years and $150,000 to just this problem, but I was also supported in this endeavor by a grant given to me after a peer review process acknowledging that this was a legitimate project.

It was during this period that I had another fortuitous meeting. I had just finished a coronary bypass graft on a middle aged man—nothing complicated, a routine procedure. It was time to wean the patient off the heart-lung bypass machine, so we could let his own heart take over pumping his blood. At this point, after taking patients off bypass, we normally use protamine to reverse the anticoagulant in the blood. Occasionally, though, there's a bad reaction and blood pressure suddenly plummets. This time the response was so severe that I had to order the perfusionist, Jery Whitworth, to put the patient back on bypass.

While waiting for the blood pressure to rise again, I stepped back from the OR table, stretched my arms, then stepped up on the little footstool we keep in the OR to see the field of operation better. From up high I peered into the chest cavity, gazing at the man's flaccid, dormant heart. Then I stepped down and muttered to no one in particular, "I knew we should have used hypnosis. He was so nervous pre-op."

"What?" said Jery from his spot at the controls of the bypass machine.

I glanced up. "You know," I said, "hypnosis . . . putting tapes on patients."

Jery rose from his knee-high stool next to the machine. "You mean using the subsconscious?" he said, suddenly excited. "Affecting blood pressure, bleeding, healing . . ."

We had caught each other's attention.

Our patient came off bypass, his heart woke up, flip-flopping back to life and a regular beat. We closed his chest, and I headed for the corridor outside the OR suites, where I collared Jery. I'd known him since I was in cardiac surgery training. An RN-turned-perfusionist in his early forties, he owned his own spread in Montana, where he once helped run a hospital. Though he was friendly and curious, we had never talked about our mutual interest in alternative healing methods.

"Hey," I said, pulling off my scrub mask, "what's your background?"

"I'm a registered nurse, a perfus—"

"No—no," I cut in, "tell me what you know about complementary medicine."

So Jery launched into a passionate recitation of his involvement in yoga, hypnotherapy, meditation, and the use of repeated, subliminal messages or words heard below a bed of music. He also told me that his interest in all this stemmed from the changes he had made in his life after the death of his father from inoperable heart disease. A postman, his father had been seemingly healthy, physically fit from walking twenty miles a day for years. But at age fifty-nine he was diagnosed a diabetic. From then on his health deteriorated dramatically, and he died.

After this very emotional period Jery, who already had a nurse's degree, studied to be a perfusionist because bypass machines made it possible for hearts to be repaired and replaced, and he wanted to be involved in cardiac care. He also deepened his knowledge of stress-reduction techniques, such as self-hypnosis and other mind-body control methods.

"You know," he said, "five or ten years ago I didn't talk about alternative medicine. I'd be labeled some kind of hippie freak. Now at least I can broach the topic."

Jery was my man. For months I had been making forays into what I preferred to call the complementary medicine field, through people like yoga teachers, massage therapists, and therapeutic-touch practitioners. But I had had a difficult time scientifically assessing these techniques. Hypnosis, I knew, was one of the most acceptable and established healing practices outside the Western norm. In psychiatry it had proven successful for decades to help curb such habits as smoking, nail biting, and overeating. Studies by such respected physicians as Harvard Medical School's Herbert Benson had shown that hypnosis can induce relaxation in heart-disease patients that has measurable therapeutic value. I reasoned hypnosis was politically the safest path to pursue for my initial studies in complementary medicine. And with Jery I had a practitioner with a solid background in scientific studies who wanted to *investigate*, not necessarily advocate, complementary medicine.

The hypnosis protocol served as the impetus to formally organize the little band of professionals interested in exploring the uses of complementary medicine at Columbia Presbyterian, including psychiatrist Stanley Fisher, resident Robbie Ashton, and an important adviser, Donald Kornfeld, a psychiatrist who was head of our Institutional Review Board, a group that had to approve all of our clinical studies. Years earlier, Don had done pioneering research in the area of post-operative patient management from a psychiatrist's perspective.

From the start I made it clear that I embraced the Western, allopathic approach to medicine, especially for treating acute illness and traumatic injuries. But for many minor, chronic, or long-term problems, other, less conventional, often simpler remedies might be called for. This was the area we would investigate. Instead of another pill for that killer migraine, perhaps an herb tea, massage, or a hypnotherapy session might bring relief without any of a drug's possible side effects. That's one of the beauties of Dr. Dean Ornish's well-known study and program to reverse heart disease naturally and without surgery. It relies on the patients' lifestyle changes, practices right from the canon of complementary healing. His program prescribes heart-healthier meals, yoga, meditation, exercise, and group-support sessions.

Our first study, which took about a year to complete and have published, focused on evaluating the role of self-hypnosis relaxation techniques on patients' pain threshold and quality of life after having coronary artery-bypass surgery. We divided patients into two randomly chosen groups, one as a control and the other as the experimental group. The night before surgery the study group was taught techniques in guided imagery aimed at relaxing muscles, lowering heart rates, and shutting out pain. The control group received no such training or treatment. At first, when we looked at the results, there appeared to be no difference between the two groups. Yet with the raw data in hand, we were able to ask another, more crucial question. Were these people doing their prescribed exercises?

Probing, we discovered only about half the hypnosis group had used the technique, and that those who used it showed less anxiety, anger, and fatigue, and didn't need as much pain medication as those who refused to perform the exercises. Almost as important, the group that had not done the exercises did worse than the patients in the control group! If nothing else, self-hypnosis gave patients a sense of participation or empowerment in their own healing. It was something they could do, could control—but only if they wanted to.

Undertaking that study helped us prepare the way to launch the department of surgery's Complementary Care Center. In Jery I found an ally who shared my vision. If he could set up the operational structure and recruit the various healers, I would design the research. I would also manage the political fallout.

I knew such an unfettered approach to the practice of medicine, even as a founding premise for a modest program in the hospital, might be incendiary. In fact, it would be difficult to get started at Columbia or any modern hospital with a reputation to protect. But I felt my colleagues would support my efforts if there were clear benefits for patients.

We procured start-up funds, got approval from the hospital, and soon opened the center for patients. Jery and I, as co-founders, had our hands more than full. I still had to be a full-time surgeon. Likewise, Jery, an organizational whiz, had his work as a perfusionist. But he ran the financial and PR side of things, while I oversaw our research and credentialing aspects in the areas of music therapy, nutrition, massage, yoga, aroma-therapy, acupressure, and therapeutic touch (or energy healing). My lab researchers would help us test each practice used.

I sometimes tell my skeptical peers that it's not so much whether this or that therapy has clearly proven clinical value, but that Americans are voting for complementary medicine with their dollars. According to a recent joint study by Boston's Beth Israel Hospital and Harvard Medical School, Americans spend about $14 billion a year on these therapies and their products, such as vitamins and herbal remedies. And most of this comes out of pocket. This figure almost matches what we spend out of pocket on all hospital admissions and is equal to the yearly cost of performing heart surgery in the United States. Moreover, in-vestigators estimate that one out of three Americans resorts to these therapies, with seven out of ten users *never* telling their personal physician about these consultations or treatments.

Once we launched our center, with its cluster of treatment rooms, offices, and waiting room, we began to make sense to many of our former detractors. Massage therapist Sarah Shaines, who also coordinates the patient-practitioner interactions, sel-dom has a shortage of patients desiring her services or wanting to sit in on the daily yoga session. "Every day I do roundups," Sarah says. "Always a lot of newcomers, a lot of people—patients and spouses—who've never tried it. Now they seek it as if it alone will save them. I just tell them it's the whole package that heals, from surgery to deep breathing."

Like Sarah, I believe that through the Complementary Care

Center I am delivering an important part of the package. Together with everything else a modern hospital offers patients—and that includes the best and latest in drugs and equipment—this comprehensive, more natural approach to healing and restored health is a true elixir. In the end patients are simply helping themselves get well.

❧ 2 ❧

Slow Down for Unicorns

Most people live, whether physically, intellectually or morally, in a very restricted circle of their potential being.

—William James

As a small boy, I had my own special paradise, a walled garden encircling my grandfather's villa on the Anatolia side of Istanbul. It was a warm, fragrant, magical place where I would spend long mornings and afternoons playing games with my younger sisters, Seval and Nazlim, or discovering the wonders of my safe little Eden. Beneath a canopy of tall shade trees, a maze of pebbled paths drew me everywhere and nowhere. Neatly trimmed hedges, higher than my head, grew along both sides of the paths, and I would lose myself in the labyrinth or emerge onto a lawn bordered by flowering shrubs, vines, and beds of lilies and roses. In the middle of it all was the garden centerpiece, a square pool of colorful mosaic tiles with a spouting fountain in the middle and clusters of goldfish drifting here and there.

To me, Turkey was a very physical world of the senses, a place and way of life that had to be seen, heard, smelled, and felt before it could be analyzed, tested, and understood. I was wrenched away from this experience after each summer vacation to return home to Delaware with my family for the school year.

Then, when I was ten, just before our usual vacation in Turkey, my father sat me down at the kitchen table. "I want you to go to my hometown," he said gravely, waiting for my reaction.

"Sure," I said.

"It's not for a day but for the whole summer," he continued. "You'll live with my oldest sister in the house where I was born."

"Baba," I said, using the affectionate Turkish word for father, "when do we go?" I was thinking of a paradise like my grandfather's villa, where I would have great adventures.

"July. You and Seval will go from Istanbul."

He made it a point that my sister and I would travel without him to the village, where our relatives would take care of us. "Nothing's really changed that much," he added. "They still sleep on a dirt floor."

I thought of camping, tents, a sleeping bag.

"Every day you sweep the dirt," he explained.

"Sweep?"

"You'll see."

From Istanbul we went to the capital city of Ankara. My aunt Ayse, a lively, motherly woman, met us there. Then she took us on a three-hour bus ride south up and down mountains to Konya, a center for the Islamic Sufi mystics and dancers. Then we rode another bus for two more hours through arid fields and rolling hills to Bozkir, my father's village, a one-road town in the hot farming belt of southern Turkey.

My aunt's two-room house, which is where my father grew up, had a dried-mud floor and a flat mud roof. There was no telephone, and a single bulb hanging from above gave us light at night. Seval and I slept on the floor in one room with our two cousins—all of us snuggled on a few blankets with a sheet pulled over the top—and my aunt and uncle slept in the other room. For a toilet we used a hole in the ground with a sewer that ran beneath it. We bathed in a tub, or at the Hamam—the Turkish bath—in the center of the village. For drinking water we went outside past the chickens and donkeys to a fountain with a spigot.

I soon loved all of it—the simple rhythm of the days, the closeness of nature and family, the sense of discovery. The only thing that gave me a problem concerned local toilet procedure. Yet this also taught me an important early lesson. Simply put, in the United States most people clean their bottoms with toilet paper. In Bozkir people wash themselves with their left hand (the right is for eating and shaking hands). The first time I stepped into their toilet room and looked at the hole in the ground with a bucket of water next to it, I was revolted. The whole business was disgusting, even barbaric, I thought.

After a few days, I brought up the subject with my relatives. "Why don't you use paper?" I asked in Turkish.

Someone spoke up. "You think wiping your rear end with toilet paper is any smarter than washing it with water?"

"Of course," I said confidently.

They then patiently explained the practical side to their argument. Paper costs money and would clog up their primitive but efficient sewer system. Also, a hand's skin and water are softer and kinder than paper, which is more abrasive and isn't as thorough. Fewer hemorrhoids, too, someone added. The clincher was the delicately posed question: "If you had some stool on your hand, would you wash it off with water, or would you wipe it off with dry paper?"

After a moment's consideration, I saw their point. And I recognized instinctively and logically that there was no right or wrong here—only different customs. I was fortunate to have had this culture-shock lesson in tolerance early in life. In shuttling back and forth between America and Turkey, I became as comfortable switching cultures as I did languages. And once medicine took over my professional life, this open-eyed view of the world allowed me to sample and examine other notions of how different people live, how they think and, of course, how they heal each other.

Even though I was still a child, I noticed a big difference between how Turks and Americans take care of their hospital patients. When I accompanied my father on visits with his former colleagues at modern clinics and hospitals in Istanbul, relatives invariably camped out day and night by the patient's bed. I'd see them giving medicines, sharing home-cooked meals, changing bed linen, and performing other simple duties. Mostly they were providing comfort, my father explained, so that the patient would never feel abandoned or alone. This was partly stimulated by inadequacies they perceived in the Turkish hospital system.

By contrast, in the U.S. hospitals where my father practiced, there were strict visiting hours, and relatives seldom if ever helped the nurses and orderlies. The hospital staff took complete charge, and visitors were usually asked to stay out of the way. Sometimes lonely faces stared at the walls or quietly filled their hours with television. I felt sorry for these people, hoping someone would appear to cheer them up. At the time I didn't think loneliness by itself could physically harm a person. But, of course, it can.

My budding awareness was furthered by the case of Bekir, the ever cheerful gardener at my grandfather's villa. At the time he was in his mid-forties, a thin, craggy-faced figure with a missing canine tooth, which was obvious because he smiled a lot. We never knew if he had been born slow or if he'd been injured in the war, but he was simple-minded. He was also deaf. Yet he was very talented at his job. Every day at dawn he would begin watering the plants, soaking the lawn and the flower beds, a happy-go-lucky presence, eagerly moving from one task to the next.

Bekir had no friends, no human contact other than with us kids and the kitchen staff, who gave him his food. His sole source of love was a stray cat and her kittens, which he cared for in his shack behind the garage. He would feed them leftover scraps from his dinner, and they slept on his bed. He would play with them, feed, and comfort them.

When my grandmother—my mother's mother—found out

about the cats, she told Bekir to get rid of them. An imperious woman, she announced the cats might be carrying diseases. But Bekir could not abandon them—he disobeyed a direct order— and one day the cats disappeared. My grandmother had them poisoned.

Within a month Bekir seemed to age a decade. No longer sunny and vibrant, he moped around the garden, sullen and lethargic. Later, after I'd returned from my summer stay in Istanbul, I heard he had become very sick and died. My mother told me that the cause of death was a "broken heart." Although I am now a cardiac surgeon and am supposed to know people don't really die of "broken hearts," I still think she was right.

I would go on to Harvard and then to medical school at the University of Pennsylvania, where my training was thoroughly Western-based, so crammed with all the basic hard science and clinical procedures a modern doctor must know that little or no attention was given to alternative healing approaches. My first task was to learn the body, and I was assigned a cadaver on the first day of my first anatomy class. I had some misgivings about making that first incision, but once I made the cut, I immediately became engrossed. Like my classmates around the big, antiseptic lab room, I stood by my table, diligently cutting, prying, opening, observing, and classifying.

I got to know "Charlie," my sixty-two-year-old cadaver, in the usual way—by identifying every possible thing inside him, from the hair follicles of his scalp to the tips of his toenails. Charlie suffered from heart disease, something I could detect from the calcified deposits of plaque in a few of his coronary arteries. I could also feel how thin the undernourished, diseased part of the heart-muscle wall was. Now limp and brownish-gray like most of his pickled body, Charlie's heart revealed little of the man beyond a pathetically abused organ. I wondered who he might have been, what kind of life would punish his heart this way. From the calluses and scars on his hands, I could tell he was probably a laborer of some kind. He was bow-legged, bald at the crown of his head, maybe twenty pounds overweight, and had a lot of cavities. Given the state of his liver, I could also tell he probably drank too much alcohol. Even though I was a medical novice, I could easily conclude that Charlie, had he taken better care of himself, could have lived a lot longer.

During that first year, anatomy as well as physiology and biochemistry absorbed me completely. Studies were a pleasure. For the first time in my life I felt that every fact, every lecture, every vein identified, was an important, relevant piece from the grand mosaic of medical knowledge. As a physician I would use it all.

On an intellectual level, I found a mechanical, physical kind of truth. But on another, more psychological level I believed I was far from enlightened. Why? Because I had encountered the "grandmother-cell theory."

If you see your grandmother on the street, I can tell you, scientifically, exactly why you recognize her shape. Your neuron networks look a bit like spindly protozoa, with cell bodies and little sharp tentacles. They touch each other, crisscrossing like electrical circuits, and combinations of these circuits play a role in producing memory. They give you an idea about shape and movement, which is always present. Even when what you see does not move, your eyeballs are always moving, fluttering. I can draw you diagrams of receptor cells, optic nerves, tracing the perception path all the way to the tiniest dendrite in a certain part of your brain. I can tell you how your eye perceives shades of dark and light on Grandma's body, on her nose, on her eyes, and on her hair. I can also explain why you discern colors. But I cannot explain how you know this blob of features is your grandmother.

Enter the grandmother-cell theory: somewhere in the billions of neurons in your brain, there is one cell that recognizes Grandma. That's its only job, to spot Grandma. When you see that certain face, hear that certain voice, notice that certain walk, you know it's Grandma.

There's no proof of this—it's just a theory we take on faith.

Yet when I finished reading this explanation by the foremost professional in the field, I could not accept it. I now know that's how medicine often works—theories fill in the blanks that can't be explained. But then I was disheartened. I felt cheated, as if I'd read a mystery story and never found out who the murderer was.

For me the grandmother-cell theory undermined the entire Western-based, allopathic system of medicine because it didn't answer the main question: How do you truly recognize Grandma? If you push the understanding of the physiological basis of medicine far enough, you'll usually come to a point that you can no longer defend it scientifically, that you must take it on faith. I couldn't.

I began to explore the possibility that there's something else that lets us recognize those we know. Call it a spiritual or unifying force that science can't yet measure or prove exists—a phenomenon somehow affected by consciousness, concern, empathy, or love. The special relationship that identical twins often have, and the many mysterious, documented cases of people who know the exact moment when something bad or good has happened to a faraway loved one. How do we explain these things without at least a glance at the non-physical qualities of the mind?

Nor are these phenomena limited to humans. In 1962, for example, researchers Sara Feather and J. B. Rhine gathered dozens of accounts about lost pets that returned to their owners from distant locales. One story that particularly impressed me was about Bobbie, a collie who was with a family traveling from Ohio to their new home in Oregon, where Bobbie had never been. At a stop in Indiana, the dog jumped out, wandered off, and apparently got lost. After unsuccessfully trying to find her, the family gave up the search and continued westward. Months later, Bobbie appeared at the new home in Oregon.

Certainly love resonates—as does rage or anxiety—prompting fluctuations in specific neurotransmitters, hormones, and various chemicals in the brain and blood. Why can't such emotions—in the form of thoughts or prayers—resonate beyond the body, reaching out around us or across great distances? Modern medicine, I concluded, would someday have to cross the chasm separating hard science and the realm of spirituality. I imagined that the human mind, body, and spirit were rays of light, intersecting somewhere inside the body. I wanted to find out where the rays fell, where the body, mind, and spirit met.

Luckily, later that year, I met the partner I would need for this quest, Lisa Lemole, my future bride. Her family and their unconventional beliefs would offer me a series of experiences and revelations that would forever change my perceptions of healing and bridge my dual cultures, East and West.

Lisa's family lived in a kind of Camelot, a hundred-acre farm just outside the Philadelphia city limits. I remember driving through the open gateway down a long driveway shaded by pine trees, passing horse paddocks, corrals, and green pastures, until I reached a large, wooden sign nailed to a tree trunk. The neatly painted black-on-white letters announced:

> *Slow down to 2 miles per hour or less*
> *Watch for children, animals,*
> *hobbits, and unicorns*
> ———
> *Violators beware of attack troll*

The Lemoles were vegetarians who lived in a small religious community called Bryn Athyn. They and most of their neighbors followed the precepts of Emanuel Swedenborg, a remarkable eighteenth-century Swedish scientist, mathematician, metallurgist, philosopher, inventor, and expert in so many other fields that he defies categorization. In his early and middle life, he made the first sketch of a glider-type airplane, and invented a submarine, a machine gun, an ear trumpet, and an airtight hot-air stove. He also discovered the function of the ductless glands and wrote the first Swedish algebra text. Then he devoted the rest of his long life until his death in 1772 to biblical interpretations that he received through visions of the eternal realm of "spirits," or angels. On one occasion Swedenborg envisioned and reported publically that Stockholm was in flames. Several days later news reached the distant town where Swedenborg lived that indeed a big fire had destroyed much of Stockholm.

Swedenborg wrote that the second coming of the Lord did not mean a return of an actual person or deity, but rather a second coming of understanding, or enlightenment about the Lord's message. He also believed that we all become angels or spirits, and that when a man and woman bond, they do so not only to become a stronger union than if each were separate and alone, but also to extend the marriage into an afterlife for eternity. The image of angels and the afterlife that has dominated Western religious art and Christian theology—both Protestant and Catholic—for the past two centuries springs in part from Swedenborg's views of this other realm.

As I began to read about Swedenborg and other works by great thinkers, I saw a central theme expressed repeatedly. Explanations of life that are based only in hard logic derived from the material world will always be insufficient; we must expand our vision to encompass additional dimensions of existence. William Blake conveyed this profound idea in simple, resonant language that I found especially moving.

> To see a World in a grain of sand,
> and a Heaven in a wild flower,
> Hold Infinity in the palm of your hand,
> And Eternity in an hour.

Lisa's father, Dr. Gerald Lemole, was a respected cardiac surgeon with sterling credentials—in 1968 he was on the world's first heart-transplant team headed by Drs. Michael De Bakey and Denton Cooley. But he also was enough of an iconoclast to prescribe vitamins for his patients long before this was fashion-able and to advocate the therapeutic benefits of massage. He theorized that by stimulating the lymphatics to eliminate toxins from the body, massage speeds healing of diseased or injured tissues—and backed up this controversial idea with data from animal experiments in which lymphatic draining was shown to increase after massaging just the foot pads of dogs.

Both he and his wife took a "holistic" view of healing, mean-ing that care of the body could not be separated from a person's emotional and spiritual life. The body and mind were one enti-ty, one whole. Mrs. Lemole, I discovered, came to this belief through a battle with Addison's disease, a rare auto-immune dis-order that affects the adrenal gland's ability to produce cortisone. During her illness she became disillusioned with the limitations of traditional medicine and started looking into such alternative healing therapies as herbs, vitamins, meditation, homeopathy, massage, and vegetarianism. Gradually she began to heal herself, using a macrobiotic diet and vitamin supplements, along with a staple treatment of cortisone, a drug that replaces a hormone that patients with Addison's lack. By the time I met her, she had long since recovered and was now thoroughly grounded in alter-native treatments that complement allopathic medicine.

In fact, she was a whiz with home remedies. For cuts, scrapes, and bruises she rubbed on calendula, a homeopathic product. For sore muscles she used arnica gel. Deeper aches and pains called for comfrey tea, an herbal remedy. For arthritic joints she suggested drinking a mixture of orange juice and cod liver oil. And she gave calcium citrate and magnesium citrate capsules for leg cramps. "These therapies often work as well as traditional Western medical remedies," she said, "so why shouldn't we use them? A simple magnesium and calcium pill can even reduce heart arrythmias. And if it doesn't work, you can still go to a doctor." She eventually convinced my father, who suffers from atrial arrythmias, to start taking calcium and magnesium supple-ments, which appeared to help his condition. And in time colleagues of mine discovered and published in respected medical journals that giving magnesium reduces the frequency of arrythmias, a complication affecting many individuals having open-heart surgery. My mother-in-law, a woman without a medical degree, was proven right.

Still, she didn't shun conventional medicine. Results were what mattered most. If the problem was acute—a broken bone, a deep cut—she was off to a hospital ER to get the bone set or the skin stitched. But for most of the common, minor ailments, from headaches, ear aches, colds, and indigestion to burns, bruises, and infections, she used her own resources. "In most cases, you can heal yourself," she likes to say. "The information's out there. You just have to look."

But at that point, a med student coming from a conservative immigrant family that believed doctors had a monopoly on good judgment, I still had a cocky, complacent attitude. Allopathic medicine would give me all the answers.

I got an important lesson in medical humility living through the birth of my first daughter, Daphne. Lisa and I were in Baltimore at a morning horse auction when her "water" broke. The amniotic fluid surrounding our first child had ruptured, and for all we knew the baby's life could be in danger. We raced back to Philadelphia, almost two hours away, to get to the midwife we had been seeing. Lisa initially had gone to an obstetrician but preferred the midwife, a woman actually recommended by the doctor when Lisa asked about this approach to delivery.

Of course, we were hoping for an uncomplicated delivery, but when we arrived at the midwife's she told us some bad news. She mentioned data from U.S. hospitals showing that once the water had broken, the fetus would become infected within twenty-four hours. Conventional practice in these cases was to induce labor if spontaneous contractions had not begun within twelve hours. About half of the women studied still could not deliver in time and required cesarean sections.

But our midwife pointed out that years ago American Indian

women of the Southwest would routinely work in the fields throughout their pregnancies, often breaking their water days before delivery.

"What happened to them?" Lisa asked.

"Nothing. They delivered healthy babies."

"No infections?"

"None, and they were never induced to premature labor."

Why? I thought. What's the difference? Was it the diet? The climate?

Our midwife had a theory. She felt that the infection of fetuses in hospitalized women was traced to health-care providers themselves, who inadvertently contaminated the women whose water had broken by doing the usual vaginal exams when checking the size of the cervix. The examiner would take his or her sterile gloved hand and slide it through the contaminated vagina and into the cervix, leaving bacteria in the previously sterile amniotic cavity.

I looked at Lisa. It was her call. From the start we had been thinking of a natural delivery, but I suspect many couples wouldn't hesitate. C-section is what conventional medicine often recommends and is responsible for saving many lives—both mother's and child's.

Lisa decided to avoid the exam and wait. I nervously paced in the hallway while she expectantly awaited the onset of contractions. Twenty-four hours later, Lisa went into labor. About thirty-six hours after her water broke, our first child came into the world without complications.*

Rather than follow the logic of conventional medicine, we had patiently waited out the process. And budding doctor that I was, I gained a deeper knowledge and a greater respect for a different approach to medical care, from a midwife armed with salves

---

*We made the decision to wait after close consultation with both our midwife and our obstetrician, who agreed that it was a rational path. I do not recommend that others in similar circumstances attempt natural childbirth without their physicians' consent.

massage techniques, and constant, savvy coaching. But I also recognized that I wanted my daughter born in a hospital where a C-section was possible—like having a safety net under the alternative approach. With this experience I felt I had entered a new frontier, one that smoothly folded old into new, making them compatible.

And a final capstone to my training would come at the end of my residency. After so many years of effort, I couldn't help but think that I had now learned the "right" way to care for patients. Then one particular baffling case brought me down to earth.

When I was called to take care of a fifty-five-year-old woman with a bleeding gastric ulcer, it seemed like a straightforward problem. She was quite sick and had bled down to a hematocrit of 17. Hematocrit is the percentage of a person's red-blood cells in the blood, which in normal people is around 45 percent. Hers was not so low that I couldn't operate, but I was upset they hadn't transfused her. Upon pursuing this "oversight," I learned that she couldn't take blood because of her religious beliefs. She was a Jehovah's Witness.

I went out to the waiting room and told the family. There must have been thirty people there, who all crowded around me. "She's going to die," I said firmly, "unless we give her blood." I explained about the low hematocrit.

We don't care—don't give her blood, the family said after conferring.

"I appreciate your religious situation," I continued. "But as her doctor, I can tell you this lady needs blood now."

"Don't give her blood," the husband repeated.

"Fine—we'll operate without it, but this is an unnecessary risk," I said, and stalked off.

Once we had her prepped in the OR, I opened her up, sewed closed the bleeding vessel in the ulcer, closed up the opening in the stomach, and brought her to the recovery room. Of course, she lost blood during the operation and from the ulcer until I got it sewn shut. Her hematocrit had dropped to 7, or so dangerously low that mostly water, not blood, was in her veins and arteries. Her undernourished organs were starting to die. She wasn't making urine, her heartbeat was irregular, her lungs were failing. She was comatose.

— I spoke to the family. "Look," I said, "healthy young people die at this hematocrit. She's not a healthy young person. She's a middle-aged woman who's bled a lot. She needs the blood."

They remained adamant in their belief.

I was perturbed at their stubbornness. "I want you to think about this carefully," I said, "because what you're telling me is that because of a religious belief you're going to kill your mom. Right?"

A few people nodded. I was perplexed. I described what would happen to her, the long, slow hours it would take for her to die. Then they asked me if they could have a little time to discuss the matter.

"All right," I said, annoyed and a touch impatient. "I'm going to make rounds and I'll be back in fifteen minutes. Discuss it, then give me your answer."

I left the room. I knew they'd change their minds. I'm a reasonably good salesman, and I'd got my point across. I figured they needed the time to let the people who were on my side convince the others that they would have to suspend the rules just this once. I instructed the nurses to get the blood ready.

"So?" I said, returning to the visiting room.

"No transfusion," a young woman said.

I was stunned. And she was not the only one who had black-balled the idea. They were uniform in their belief. I was so angry, I left the hospital. I couldn't stand to see her die. I couldn't believe they would, in effect, kill her. She was *my* patient. I went home, leaving junior residents to oversee her demise. I was done with the case; I was powerless to save her from her misguided relatives.

She hung on during the first evening, then through the next day, and into the next week. Every hour she improved. Somehow she managed to survive with practically no blood in her body. And in a couple of days her bone marrow revved up and started making new blood. Within a week she already had a blood count of 12. She continued to make new cells and eventually climbed back to a safe count. In less than two weeks she went home.

Her survival humbled my professional pride. Dr. Hard Science was wrong. I had been thinking so much of my own success as a doctor that I missed what was really going on. Eventually I puzzled it out. I had disregarded the family's wishes because I didn't understand what they were saying. They didn't say, "Don't transfuse because we think she's going to live." They said, "Don't do it because we think it's the right thing to do. If her time's up, it's up. If not, she'll live."

Today I still would prefer to talk my patients into receiving blood if it's needed. I strongly feel that religious rules requesting medical care that has unclear foundations should not be blindly adhered to by patient or family. However, I can understand that for people like the family of my patient, there was a goal held higher than living the next day. If I'd given the woman a transfusion and she had lived, I would have gone against everything she thought sacred. Her family understood that; I did not. Their attitude allowed me to see another, more spiritual dimension to recovery. Maybe their prayers worked. Maybe some other dynamic we can't yet understand in scientific terms was involved.

I, the doctor, did *not* always know best. I had my limitations. It was the best lesson I could have learned at the time. The survival of my Jehovah's Witness patient catalyzed my pursuit of treatments beyond the conventional. Again, but now from a different position, I began to open my eyes to a much wider view of healing and health care. The results would be revolutionary—for myself and for my patients.

❧ 3 ❧

High Tech, No Tech

The patient's hopes are the physician's best ally.

—Norman Cousins

Welcome to the twenty-first century, the age of the high-tech fix. The average person comes to us believing hard science and modern medicine will fix almost any problem. So we tally the symptoms, do all the measurements and tests—efficiently and scientifically—with all our electronic monitors, X rays, and lab tests to get clear-cut results.

But the correct diagnosis we're seeking depends on more than mere test data. We have to consider all the factors contributing to the condition. Take coronary-artery disease, for example. Not all heart-disease patients understand that they belong to a very diverse group of people, each with a different set of factors contributing to his or her problem. Some have all the risk factors—the patient is a smoker, he's fat, eats all the wrong foods, doesn't exercise, has a high cholesterol level and a family history of heart attacks. Then there's the person who *shouldn't* have heart disease—the woman is slim, eats right, doesn't smoke, jogs, and her parents have no heart problems. But contrary to what might be predicted from these factors, the obese man lives on with his clogged coronaries, and the slender woman has a massive heart attack.

What's going on? Checking further, we might discover that the fat man, who looks like a cardiac time bomb, has a gentle, jolly temperament that is unlikely to send his coronaries into potentially deadly spasms. As for the lady, we might find that her husband had left her or was having an affair, and that this betrayal and her subsequent depression damaged her heart.

There's no question that a person's emotional life can affect the heart. A good example is one of my patients, John Haelin, a seventy-year-old caterer from upstate New York. He dieted and exercised regularly. He had never suffered any serious injury or illness, nor had he ever been hospitalized. The active father of eight grown children, John liked to play golf and ski, and was blessed with a sunny, even temperament. Certainly he was not the typical candidate for a heart attack.

But one night he had been awakened by a loud crashing at the front of his house. Before he could sit up, two large men burst into his bedroom. Both figures lunged across the room and, tearing off his blankets, began beating him, striking him repeatedly in the face. John tried futilely to protect himself with his hands until one of the men grabbed the phone and, bashing him over the head, knocked him unconscious.

When the paramedics arrived, they found John bleeding and moaning. At the hospital, doctors treated his broken nose, cuts, and bruises, and monitored his concussion and double vision. Then surgeons repaired his left eye socket and cheekbone by inserting a titanium plate. After ten days in the hospital, he was finally discharged—a physically and emotionally broken man.

"I felt violated, completely helpless," John told me months later at Columbia. "There's nothing worse."

Eight months after the assault, for which the culprits were arrested and prosecuted, John was again attacked—this time from within his own body, by angina.

"It didn't happen overnight," John said, "but I was slowing down. I kept thinking it was because I was getting older."

He'd begun to feel a tightness in his chest that made breathing difficult. His personality had also changed, and he'd grown fearful, withdrawn, emotionally spent. By the time I saw John, instead of looking like a virile seventy going on fifty, he was a sedentary, lethargic seventy-year-old who looked eighty.

After listening to John's account of the beating, I could track the clear downward spiral that had finally pushed him to seek help. Luckily his early-warning system of telltale symptoms—energy drain, tightening chest pressure, and breathing trouble—kept him from experiencing the walloping pain of the classic heart attack victim. But he could easily have joined the army of unfortunates who die every day of the big one—"MI" or heart attack. About one-third of all MI victims die, making it the biggest killer in the Western world.

Even a long-buried trauma can seriously affect a person's health. One of my colleagues, Dr. Samuel Mann of Cornell Medical Center's New York Hospital, had a patient who was severely hypertensive. Both her parents and her sisters were hypertensive, and her mother had died at age forty-three of the condition. But Dr. Mann's patient had been living contentedly for many years with a male companion. She did clerical work, which she enjoyed, didn't smoke or drink alcohol, and reported no particular stress in her life. Given her lifestyle, despite her genetic predisposition, she shouldn't have had blood pressure that was so out of control. She was taking five medications, but her pressure stayed in the range of 150 to 170 over 120 to 130 mm Hg. She had periods of speech loss, had already undergone surgery for a clogged artery, and was suffering from several other cardiovascular-related problems.

Then, during a routine visit to her doctor, she complained of a recurring nightmare in which a man would attack her from behind, grabbing her and pushing her down. Each time she had the dream she would wake up screaming, "He hurt me. He hurt me."

She was now afraid to go to bed or go to sleep. When questioned she revealed—for the first time in thirty years—that she had been raped at age fourteen by her sister's fiancé. She had been hospitalized for two weeks with a pelvic infection that left her infertile, but still she kept the rape secret to avoid destroying her family.

After she disclosed the rape, the patient's pressure rose to 240 over 150, then began to decrease. By the next day it was down to a more normal 120 over 85. She soon began counseling sessions, and her life brightened dramatically. Though she must still take medications to control what is a familial condition, her hypertension is now quite manageable.

I put LVADs into patients with the expectation that the procedure will restore them to health. But some recovering patients, who I've felt should have been happy to be alive, have wanted more and remained in the doldrums. So, from my earliest years as a surgeon, I have been forced to confront the difference between health and lack of disease.

I had one patient with such a sense of self-blame for his heart attack that I believe it nearly killed him. I had put a new heart in him, but his body immediately rejected it. Each day he grew progressively sicker. When I told him that he was rejecting and needed another operation, this big, strong fellow broke down and cried. I discovered in talking to him that he hated his new heart. He felt that his old one had abandoned him and blamed himself for all his complications. Weighed down by guilt, he felt that the new heart was back-stabbing him.

Now, if you think your heart is fighting you, then you're battling a civil war with your body and you can't move ahead toward healing. We turned things around physically for this patient by removing fluid from around his heart and adjusting his immunotherapy, but not until he could accept that it was his depression, not his heart, that was the problem could he make a real commitment to recovery.

Since most heart-disease patients have to remain at the hospital for months, they are especially vulnerable to severe depression, which can be lethal. Patients know that they have almost died. They have faced their own mortality, and for some it has been a terrifying experience. The heart-lung machine itself may also affect the chemical balance of the brain and induce a biochemical depression. Then there's the lingering prospect that the same conditions that prompted the original heart attack may be waiting in the wings, ready to cause another.

Various studies, of course, strongly suggest that depression and heart disease are somehow connected. For example, in one eighteen-month Canadian study of 222 heart-attack patients, depression was found to be a significant predictor of post-operative mortality among the 19 who died from cardiac causes. Carried out by the Montreal Heart Institute, the study also linked post-operative deaths to major depression and depressive symptoms while in hospital care.

Another study, begun in the early 1980s by Dr. William W. Eaton of the Johns Hopkins School of Hygiene and Public Health, traced more than 1,500 people in the general population thirteen years after they had been screened for depression. As with any cross section of people, some were depressives and others were not; some had heart attacks while others didn't. When Dr. Eaton and his researchers adjusted their data to account for such factors as age, sex, marital status, and high blood-pressure history, they found that people who suffered depressions were four times as likely to have a heart attack.

Though medical researchers still don't know for certain whether depression promotes heart disease or vice versa, some have discovered physiological changes that occur with depression—such as higher levels of stress hormones. Dr. Richard Veith, a professor of psychiatry and behavioral science at the University of Washington in Seattle, for instance, found that levels of norepinephrine in the blood of depressed patients are 30 percent higher than in the blood of non-depressed patients. This hormone speeds up the heart rate and raises blood pressure, which increases the workload on the heart and, if coronary arteries are already narrowed, the risk of an attack.

Early in my practice I found—and many surgeons would concur—that if a critically ill person doesn't want to live, he or she often dies on the OR table or in the intensive care unit. Two of my own patients taught me the importance of an elemental, often overlooked factor in sustaining life: the human spirit.

Harry Leasure and Nigel Peterson were practically bookend cases. Both were in their fifties, both had seriously impaired hearts, and both entered the ICU around the same time. After they received left ventricular-assist devices, both were put on the transplant list, and both had similar significant post-operative complications.

When I first saw Harry Leasure, he was in the intensive care unit, hooked up to the usual monitors and breathing with the help of a respirator. I had been brought in on his case because he was considered a possible LVAD candidate. I looked at his chart and checked the various monitors. "He's not fully brain dead," the neurologist later told me outside Harry's room, "but it's so much that I think it's irreversible."

"Then there's not much to do," I said. "We watch and wait."

Harry, I learned, had suffered a mild heart attack about fifteen years ago, then recovered without surgery with the usual regimen of low-fat diet, moderate exercise, and medication. Now he had come in with an irregular heart rhythm, followed four days later by a massive cardiac arrest, which in turn cut off blood to his brain. From what we observed and what neurological tests showed, the blood-flow interruption had caused a swelling of brain tissues from the lack of oxygen. Aside from these medical facts and that he ran the operations of a large New Jersey bus company, I knew little about the man. The rest I would learn from his wife, Sandy.

I met her briefly in the visitors lounge and after that would usually find her in Harry's room by his bed. She was trim, pretty, and maybe twenty years younger than her husband, who despite his moribund appearance was a compact, robust fellow with a broad, handsome face. "His body looks in pretty good physical shape," I told her just after we met. She explained he was very active at work but never really exercised for fitness or played a sport like golf or tennis. "Maybe a little bowling," Sandy said, "but that's about it." She also mentioned walking around a lot on cruise ships. They had been in the Caribbean not long before his latest heart woes began, and she thought that maybe all the rich food on board had worsened his heart condition.

She might have been correct, but more than likely a combination of factors going as far back as his birth and genetic makeup had led Harry to his present condition. A family predisposition for heart disease, temperament, diet, weight, cigarette smoking, and a lack of exercise—all contribute to the buildup of fatty deposits in and on the walls of coronary arteries. How did he live his life? How did he handle problems, crises, anger? I didn't know. But whatever fated him to be here, like nearly all my patients, Harry was very sick.

"How are you doing?" I asked Sandy.

"I'll be okay—once he gets better."

Harry's condition had deteriorated beyond what a coronary surgery bypass graft could remedy. His damaged heart muscle was functioning at ten percent of normal. In fact, nothing of permanent use could be done for him until he showed signs of coming to his senses, of reviving neurologically. Then I might consider giving him an LVAD pump so he could stay alive while waiting for a donor heart.

I told Sandy the neurologist had suggested Harry would probably never be what he was before because of the injury to his brain. A lot of memory might be lost. There was the possibility of his remaining comatose. "He'll wake up," she said, shaking her head confidently. "He just needs somebody to help him."

By the time I see patients, being a cardiothoracic surgeon, they've usually been seen by their personal physician, their cardiologist, and maybe several other specialists. They've been tested, medicated, blitzed with needles, IV lines, and catheter tubes. Their families are all too familiar with doctors, nurses, orderlies, long waits, hospital food, our procedures, and even our jargon: *immunosuppressive* for the drugs that minimize organ-transplant rejection, *tachycardia* for rapid heart beat, and *cabbage* for CABG, or coronary artery bypass graft.

So, whenever possible, my approach to family members is upbeat and positive. I want them to believe that as long as their loved one is alive, he or she has a chance. Even when I'm faced with what I think are hopeless or near-hopeless cases, I try to offer some notion that there's a light ahead, a way out of the nightmare. Such encouragement sometimes helps relatives take a more determined, positive attitude toward their loved one's plight. It's an intangible factor, but one that can often affect a patient in subtle ways—before, during, and after surgery.

Though Harry's situation was grim, I told Sandy he just might rally. When she answered with such clear-eyed confidence that she would help bring him back, I was surprised but pleased, since patient relatives are often too scared, worried, or emotionally upset to make such pronouncements. True to her word, she stayed by her husband's bed, from seven in the morning until late at night. Thirty miles home, then back again the next morning. Whenever I'd drop by to check on Harry, I'd see her talking and whispering to him, kissing him on the forehead and holding his hand. For three days she carried on a continuous one-sided conversation. I noticed she wore a thin necklace with a small gold cross. She told me it was something her mother gave her and that she never took off. "I say all my prayers with it," she said.

On the fourth day, I held Harry's hand and told him to squeeze it. Earlier, Sandy said she had felt movement, but I wasn't getting a response. "You try," I told her.

She moved in and raised his hand in hers. "Come on, honey," she said. "Squeeze my hand, give me a sign."

I waited as she continued to coax him. If he moved even one

finger, I thought it would be miraculous. If her words penetrated and he understood, he'd have to make a Herculean effort to respond. He wasn't even breathing on his own, had no control of bodily functions, was practically comatose, and here we were, expecting him to give the okay sign. I wasn't optimistic. Then suddenly Sandy said, "Look, he moved a finger!"

At first I saw nothing. His hand looked as lifeless as before. But then I thought I saw an almost imperceptible quiver of his middle and index fingers. Had he moved them or was it my imagination? I watched closely and concluded Harry indeed had moved two fingers. By the next day he had clearly awakened from his coma.

The team decided to go ahead and give him a chance. I took him to the OR and, without major complications, inserted an LVAD pump into him. The surgery went quite smoothly. Still, out of habit, I remained wary. I've seen too many unexpected reversals to be complacent even after the most trouble-free surgeries.

Sure enough, when we got Harry back to his recovery room, the rhythm of his heartbeat suddenly went berserk. Then there was no beat at all, no blood being pushed to Harry's brain. He would be dead within five minutes. I began compressing his chest, pushing down on his heart with my hands to temporarily keep blood circulating in his body. Finally, I brought him back, using the defibrillation paddles, then altering his IV-drip medications. We'd entered the eye of the storm. I whisked him to the OR again and connected his right ventricle to a second assist-device pump. He now had an LVAD for the left side of his heart, and an RVAD for the right side.

Sometimes in medicine we say, "The operation was a success, but the patient died." Harry seemed to be approaching this kind of grim "success."

Back with him in the ICU recovery room, I considered the probable damage to his brain. He had now survived two periods when the blood supply was cut off. Both episodes had to have been severely traumatic. Other consulting doctors offered pessimistic views, giving Harry a bleak prognosis. This time when I spoke to Sandy, I had trouble sounding positive, but I did my best to raise her spirits. I praised her round-the-clock attentions to Harry and told her I was hoping he would eventually pull through.

Victory over illness often requires more than smarts and stamina. It also takes a determined attitude, a stubborn will to prevail. All his life Harry had been a go-getter, a self-made guy who rose from driving a bus to running the whole bus company. But here he was, slipping helplessly toward death.

One evening while I was doing late rounds, I spotted Sandy at her usual place. "What's up?" I said, approaching Harry's bed. I glanced at a few monitors; his signs looked about the same as the last time I was by.

"He's squeezing my fingers again," Sandy said.

She called it squeezing, probably because she could feel a tiny movement of his fingers in her hand. But when I stared down at Harry's arm, focusing intently on those five pale digits, I couldn't really tell if he had moved them.

"Great," I said, then suggested she get some sleep. Keeping the other caregivers healthy is an important task of a healer.

"No way," she said. "I can't leave now. Harry might wake up."

"What makes you think he'll wake up now and not tomorrow?"

"Because a little while ago he fluttered his eyelids. I saw them, I felt them."

I bent closer and noticed the minute stirrings under his eyelids. Those tiny movements and twitches of an awakening mind connected to a body continued for a few more days, until Harry opened his eyes. More time passed, and soon he began to mumble, then talk. Finally, slowly, he began to answer questions. I told Sandy that she should insist that his mind stay active and in contact with what was going on around him. She read him newspaper stories, cajoled him into simple responses, helped him search for words. Harry somehow mastered his frustration and agitation—I never had to order him restrained as I did other disoriented, brain-impaired patients—and gradually he regained his mind, recovered his humanity.

How had he recovered?

During his illness parts of Harry's brain had been temporarily damaged. Brain cells, called neurons, are connected to each other by threadlike appendages—dendrites and axons—through which messages are sent and received. When a brain cell is stimulated, an electrical impulse triggers the release of chemicals called neurotransmitters, which jump across a microscopic gap called a synapse to the receiver cell or neuron. The more connections made, the greater the growth of dendrites. In Harry's brain these networks of neurons were most likely distorted or disconnected.

Recent neurological research suggests that stimulating the mind, as Sandy did with her words and touch, can spur neurons to grow and branch out like the roots of a growing tree. This branching creates more connections between the neurons. This is how memory is built and enhanced in billions of brain cells, created essentially by a patient's interaction with others, not by machines or drugs. Sandy helped her husband build new connections to reconstruct his memory. Her attentions and presence were Harry's best mind therapy, which of course helped his body.

Sandy never lost confidence that she could help him retrieve his mind. It wasn't that she knew this medically; she knew this viscerally. "I had no choice," she told me. On the day he got his new heart, Sandy wrote:

Wednesday:

Transplant team calls me 2 a.m. to tell me they have a heart for you and they want permission to go ahead. I come about 3 or 4 o'clock. They take you into the operating room. Dr. Oz comes out to the waiting room at 6:30 to see me, to tell me the donor heart arrived. It looked good and he's going ahead with the surgery.

He came back out to me at 9 a.m. and said it was all finished and there were no more pumps or anything in you. When I went in to see you, it was so quiet. No more pumping. No more machines or anything. Just you.

Nigel Peterson also came to the hospital as a place of last resort. An international businessman from Trinidad, he wore a permanent frown, looking irritated at the whole business of ICU attentions—the intravenous drips, the tangle of electrode wires sprouting here and there around his chest, the respirator mask, all the monitors and the various strange people bustling in and out of the room. Unlike most patients—who are cooperative and submit to such activity without much fuss—Nigel wanted none of it.

Yet he needed us and our machines and medicines if he was to survive. Five years before, one of my colleagues had performed a high-risk, quadruple bypass operation on him. At the time Nigel suffered from diabetes, had a high cholesterol level, smoked cigarettes, and drank too much alcohol. After the operation he quit the bad habits and seemed to do fine for a few years. Now he was back in the hospital with odd, atypical pains, occurring sporadically in different parts of his chest. His blood pressure was nose-diving, and his heart's ejection fraction had dropped to a dangerously low 12, which meant that his heart was pumping blood out to the body at only 12 percent of its normal force. Not enough oxygenated blood was nourishing his brain. Mr. Peterson was in "extremis"—our shorthand for someone near death.

The consult team—those observing and treating him— quickly huddled. Since I would do the operation, it was my call. I decided he was a good enough candidate for an LVAD pump, but the social worker objected. "I don't see much family support," she said. "Where are the relatives? Who's going to watch out for him, take him home, bring him in?"

I learned Nigel was married, though I never saw visitors in his room, not even his wife. Whenever I examined him, he appeared aloof, even arrogant, and revealed little of himself. As with most heart-disease patients, Nigel's present crisis was only the tip of the iceberg. Serious stress of some sort helped break him. Whatever the cause, he was retreating into a mood of isolation and deep depression.

We took him to the OR. By the time I donned my surgical gown, gloves, and jeweler-like head loupes that magnify my work area, the surgical team had him prepped and anesthetized, waiting for me to make that first slice into the skin over the chest. As soon as I sawed through the sternum, spreading apart the chest bone for a look at my target, I knew I was in for a very difficult operation—a ten-straight-hour procedure as it turned out.

The pericardial sac was stuck fast to the heart. Normally this enveloping membrane peels away without too much cutting needed. With Nigel Peterson, who had layers of scar tissue built up under the sac, it was like carving into marble—chip here, chip there. The movements of my fingers had to be tiny, discreet, and very tedious. Slice, cut, trim, stab—all within the confines of a cavity the size of my ten-year-old daughter's sneaker. Once I exposed the heart, I had to contend with bleeding on practically every surface—the cut sternum bone, the sliced-through skin and muscle edges, the heart muscle, the scar tissue.

It was finger-in-dike time, except there seemed to be hundreds of holes. Nigel's blood had no clotting factors because of his dysfunctional liver and kidneys. Blood was backing up into the liver and preventing it from making clotting factors. Blood was also backing up into the kidneys, so he wasn't making urine. No sooner had I cauterized and stanched one little flood than three or four other bleeders burst out. By the time the torrent slowed and we had him in a recovery room, he was still bleeding a liter every hour.

We waited. In the recovery room I opened him again, found more bleeders and stopped them. After twenty-four hours of struggle, the oozing stopped, the LVAD whooshed along with metronomic regularity, and my patient's heart, even his liver, started to recover.

But his kidneys didn't, and most important, neither did his brain. For three weeks we tended to him in recovery. Throughout this time he remained disoriented, depressed, lethargic; he grew frustrated, became agitated, and we had to keep him strapped down in bed to keep him from possibly removing necessary intravenous lines, various monitor wires and tubes. But I was still hopeful. When lucid, Mr. Peterson could follow simple commands. I remember asking him the classic three questions. "Who are you?" I began.

The frail dark-skinned figure hesitated, then whispered his name.

"Where are you?"

He glanced around, cleared his throat, and haltingly announced, "Hospital."

"When did you come here?"

For a moment he gazed at me as if he didn't understand the question. I repeated it, trying to coax a date or time from a memory probably battered by one too many mini-strokes. Silence. He would not answer. Then slowly he began to shut down. His eyes went blank and he lost all expression. His head seemed to disappear into the pillow. From a conscious, living person he melted away.

Over the next few days I realized Nigel Peterson would not play a role in making himself better. He didn't have the strength or the desire. I did all I could for him as a scientist, and since he had no other visitors others on the staff spent a lot of time with him. But my medical training had not included ways to help such a patient bolster this critical quality—the grit and determination to hang on to life.

After three weeks of struggle, Mr. Peterson's liver, lungs, and kidneys failed; infections finally took over. His body was irreversibly injured, and he was in a coma. Finally I had no choice but to turn off the pump and let him die with dignity.

Why did Nigel Peterson die and Harry Leasure live? In some respects, Harry was actually worse off. Unlike Nigel, Harry's crippled heart had diminished the functioning of his brain for weeks, yet he came back. We then did the transplant, and he eventually made a near-complete recovery. On a purely physiological level, such a recovery didn't make sense.

The only big difference between the two cases was one of spirit. Harry had Sandy at his side; Nigel had no one. Nigel might have lived if he hadn't been so lonely. He desperately needed emotional companionship, pep talks, someone to coax back his will to live. How could he harness his own powers to heal himself if there was no one to calm him down, comfort him, hold his hand, or encourage him?

We all know that the loss of a family member can cause the death of a close relative. I have a vivid picture of a depressed, eighty-two-year-old Italian man whose heart and other organs were finally giving up on him. His wife, who was in her seventies, was a small, excitable woman who had been married to him for more than fifty years and was now very upset that her husband said he wanted to die. I told her my biggest fear was that she wouldn't be able to cope with his dying. I reminded her that she had children and grandchildren to live for. I thought I had calmed her down, but as she and some of her family members left my office, she passed out in the hallway and I had to rush out to resuscitate her.

When she came to, I reminded her, "I just told you not to do that. That's exactly the kind of thing that's going to kill you." Then I had her sit down, close her eyes, and think about someplace nice. Her blood pressure, which had just shot up to a dangerous 220 over 110, came down to 170 over 100. I turned down the lights and told her to keep thinking pleasant thoughts.

In ten minutes her numbers were down to a more normal 130 over 80.

The reason her husband—a high-risk candidate for a coronary-bypass operation—was dying was unclear. What was clear was his desire to die. With an exhausted, haunted look about him, he simply moved his head from side to side, then whispered, "I can't go on. I'm done." I tried to cheer him, but he closed his eyes and repeated, "I'm done, I don't care. I want to die."

And he did. There was nothing we could do. His loving, seemingly healthy wife died soon thereafter, apparently determined to follow her husband in leaving this world. This is a commonly reported occurrence, especially among lifelong partners who both figuratively and literally cannot live without each other.

Given today's tremendous demand for our medical services, few doctors and even fewer surgeons are ever able to study individual patients this closely or this well. I was lucky to have learned from cases like those of Nigel Peterson and Harry Leasure.

So I pursued my discovery a bit further, mostly to satisfy my very Western hunger for hard scientific data to support what I had witnessed. What occurs biochemically when a very sick, unconscious person is lured awake by a loved one's comforting words and caresses?

Rigorous research by Candace Pert, a neurological scientist at Georgetown University, and others point to the curative role of certain chemicals regulating brain—and consequently body— function. These chemicals are neuropeptides, or strings of amino acids made by nerve and glial cells, named after the Greek word for glue. Glial cells form a kind of nourishing honeycomb that protects the brain cells. When these neuropeptides connect to receptors attached to other cells in the body—including immune cells—they cause physical reactions. Dr. Pert has shown that neuropeptides and their receptors form an information network the body uses to communicate with itself. She believes this network is the biochemical substrate, or form, of emotions—something like the circuitry that controls the body's ability to fight an attacker or flee from danger. In the case of neuropeptides, the circuitry that enables them to flow throughout the body scientifically explains how the mind can promote the healing of the body.

But Dr. Pert cautions that we shouldn't think of it solely as a brain-centered system: emotions are not only in the head; she believes there's also a cellular consciousness and that every cell has receptors and a "wisdom" of its own. Thus, a bone cell functions differently from a liver cell. All cells might be said to "know" what each is supposed to do, independent of messages from the brain.

Dr. Pert concludes that feelings, or emotional energy, come first; then the peptides are released throughout the body. So consciousness precedes matter. For example, when we do deep breathing in yoga exercises, we're consciously changing the release of peptides in the body. We are changing, perhaps energizing or relaxing, our emotional state. In this way our very breath can be an ally in healing.

Other scientists in the relatively new field of psychoneuroimmunology have discovered overwhelming evidence that our minds and emotions affect our immune systems. We also know that depression, loneliness, or such stressful blows as a loved one's death, a divorce, or the loss of our job lowers immunity against disease. More than this—specifically what we know about *how* this happens in our brains and bodies—is still being pursued in labs and research centers around the world.

My experience with patients like Harry Leasure and Nigel Peterson increasingly drew my attention not only to the biochemical reasons behind emotions, but also to social aspects involved. Apart from the many studies strongly linking depression, smoking, overweight, and inactivity to heart disease, research was providing convincing data that such factors as friendships, jobs, particular workdays, and time of day play a role in producing heart attacks. As noted earlier, one ten-year study of 2,254 cardiac-care patients found that more fatal cardiac arrests occur on Monday and Saturday than on any other day of the week. Investigators at Leicester General Hospital in England explained that Mondays and Saturdays, especially for men, were days on which people must adjust to a new routine or phase, whether of work or of leisure. Apparently, the stress of returning to work or to a crammed weekend of home chores, errands, hobbies, and social obligations may induce a heart attack.

Researchers at New York Hospital also studied several hundred employed men, from thirty to sixty years of age, and concluded that higher demands and less control at work may create enough "job strain" to produce hypertension and a larger, less efficient heart. Thus, an assembly-line worker doing quick, repetitive tasks with low levels of control over the process endures more stress than his manager, who has more control and autonomy.

I was also impressed with studies suggesting that having close friends may promote all-around good health more than living a virtually friendless existence. After all, we have evolved as social beings, and such gestures as shaking another's hand, hugging, and kissing have definite neural and hormonal consequences, all potentially helpful to the heart. Anxiety or anger can change our breathing, tense our muscles, make us perspire, race our heart, and dilate our pupils. Conversely, an embrace can slow our breathing, relax our muscles, ease the heartbeat, and soften the eyes.

I didn't need piles of studies to convince me that my patients in particular and Western medicine in general could benefit from some of the more proven and promising modalities of complementary medicine. What led me to this gradual turning point in my career I owe to my dual-culture childhood and schooling— one steeped in ancient, central Asian ways, and the other in modern, Western science. When I performed surgery on doomed

Nigel Peterson, I tried to save his life with my skills. But I also felt he could have been helped by the kind of comfort Sandy Leasure gave to her husband. I felt helpless when Mr. Peterson died. Long before and after surgery, I should have paid more attention to his emotional status.

His case was an indelible lesson, though I might not have come to this conclusion if I hadn't had a long string of such lessons—small and large discoveries that began in early childhood. As I remember, one of my first revelations on my journey to become a healer occurred in the sunburnt desert town of Burdar in southern Turkey.

4

Crusoe Calls

Imagery, as we use it, is another way to harness the extraordinary power of your mind.

—Dr. Herbert Benson

Because my parents were Turkish-born, I had dual Turkish-American citizenship. But to continue my Turkish rights—including the right to inherit property and even visit Turkey—I needed to complete basic training in the Turkish military. When I arrived at our boot camp in Burdar, I felt as if I had walked into an oven. A few pine trees and scrub brush dotted the surrounding plain, which was a virtual desert. Rock, sand, sun, and little else but heat waves appeared in the distance.

Every morning our routine was the same. Decked out in our woollen uniforms, we bald-headed recruits were lined up and ordered to march in precise military formations, with brisk high-kicking, goose-stepping strides. That done, we returned to camp and had to stand perfectly still at attention for endless periods in the oppressive heat. "No one moves!" the gruff captain would shout. "Not a twitch!"

The first time I went through this endurance exercise, I didn't know if I would last. If only there was a breeze, I thought, straining to feel just a breath of desert air. Nothing. But then I closed my eyes and blew upward across my face, simulating a cooling effect. I kept blowing, imagining a strong cool gust arising from the northern plains of the Crimea and the Black Sea, and driving straight into my face. As I concentrated, focusing my thoughts on coolness, I pictured being on the bow of a sailboat on the Bosporus, with the sea wind and cold, refreshing spray whipping over my face and body. And I actually grew chilled—so much so that I could feel goose bumps prickling down my back.

Nothing around me had changed. The sun was just as hot, but somehow I'd lowered my body temperature. I'd already had a few years of medical training, so I could analyze the physical aspects of what had occurred. By closing my eyes and concentrating on a cooling scene, I had entered a hypnotic state. This affected my autonomic nervous system—the autopilot system of the body—and my heart rate probably dropped and I stopped sweating. Physiologically my body had been changed by my mind.

Herbert Benson, author and pioneer in mind-body research at Harvard Medical School, studied what happens to people when they elicit the physiological changes of the "relaxation response," which he contrasts with the well-known, adrenaline-pumping, fight-or-flight response. Dr. Benson and his colleagues found that when subjects assumed relaxed positions in a quiet setting, closed their eyes, and concentrated on repeating certain thoughts or images, they significantly lowered their oxygen intake, heart rate, blood pressure, and respiratory rate. In his bestselling book, *The Relaxation Response*, Dr. Benson holds that to enter such a state, passively ignoring distracting thoughts, certain repetitive techniques are commonly used, such as meditation, repeated prayers, yoga stretching, deep, diaphragm breathing, and imaging or visualizing. Under the intense Turkish sun during my military boot camp, I must have elicited my relaxation response.

Many well-documented cases of ascetic wise men in India and elsewhere demonstrate far more amazing feats of endurance while in similar hypnotic-like states. A yogi in Tibet, for example, can reduce his heart rate to ten beats per minute. Nearly naked yogin are able to stay outside in freezing weather for hours and never become hypothermic. Then there are the men and women of various traditional cultures who can safely walk barefoot over burning coals.

Even in the West for centuries some dentists and physicians have used hypnosis to block their patients' perception of pain when undergoing tooth extractions and minor surgery, and there are cases on record of hypnotized women delivering babies virtually "pain-free" by cesarean section. Many people also use self-hypnosis to manage such day-to-day problems as stress, anxiety, migraines, irritable bowel syndrome, obesity, and nail biting, smoking, and other addictions.

The word *hypnosis* is derived from the name of the Greek god of sleep, Hypnos. But unlike a sleeping person, someone in a trancelike, hypnotic state is quite alert and in control of his or her actions. It's a voluntary process. Most people remain awake, and many continue to hear everything around them, which is hardly like true sleep. A hypnotized person shifts from analytic to synesthetic thinking—that is, the mind depends less on logic and more on sensations and feelings. This more free-flowing state of mind is often described as the trance state.

Today, hypnotherapy, or the formal, medical use of hypnosis, is one of the most scientifically endorsed complementary therapies. As an aid in surgery and recovery, hypnosis has been shown to have definite therapeutic benefits. Scientists led by Marcia Greenleaf and Stanley Fisher at the Albert Einstein College of Medicine in New York, for example, demonstrated this in a study on the effects hypnosis had on thirty-two coronary-bypass patients. Some were taught self-hypnosis with imagery for muscle relaxation, while other, control-group patients received no training.

The self-hypnosis training was given to two groups in forty-five-minute sessions one to two days before surgery. As the investigators describe it, for a patient to enter into a trance, a three-step procedure should be followed:

At *one:* You look up as if you are trying to look up
toward the top of your head. Do it now. . . . That's
right.

At *two:* Keep looking up, and as you keep looking up,
close your eyes slowly. That's right. As you keep
looking up, take a deep breath. Hold it for the count
of three . . . 1-2-3.

At *three:* Exhale, let your eyes relax, and just let your
body float.

To bring yourself out of trance, use a three-step procedure. Count backward from three to one.

At *three:* Get ready. Do it now.

At *two:* With your eyes still closed, look all the way up.

At *one:* Open your eyes slowly, permitting them to
come into focus.

In one group patients in trance were taught simply to relax,
imagining themselves as limp and floppy rag dolls or bean bags.
They were instructed that holding these thoughts in mind would
allow muscle relaxation in every part of the body. In the second
group patients in trance were given specific suggestions to help
themselves by mentally focusing on doing six things: (1) letting
their bodies know how to respond before, during, and after
surgery; (2) letting their defense systems stay alert during surgery
to protect themselves; (3) cooperating with treatment by flowing
along with the procedures; (4) having a clean, dry wound and
minimal bleeding and discomfort; (5) keeping their blood pressure comfortable; and (6) looking forward to a quick return to
thirst, appetite, moving about, and ease of toilet visits. These patients were also told to focus on returning to a lifestyle free of
pain and fear.

Investigators monitoring the three groups measured such
physiological effects as blood pressure, wound drainage, and
length of time on a respirator and concluded that the degree of a
patient's susceptibility to hypnosis was a significant predictor of

stability in post-operative recovery from major surgery. Patients who were in the mid-range of "hypnotizability"—regardless of which self-hypnosis group they were in—recovered faster in the first forty-eight hours after surgery than the other patients. The researchers also speculated that it might be possible to fine tune suggestions and instructions, depending on each patient's particular problems and capacity to be hypnotized.

At our Complementary Care Center, we completed a similar trial with thirty-five cardiac patients. As with the Greenleaf-Fisher study, we selected our patients on a random basis, but divided them into two groups instead of three: those who were hypnotized and taught self-hypnosis techniques and those who were not hypnotized. We found that patients taught self-hypnosis had lower scores for fatigue, while those who were taught hypnosis but didn't follow through on the proper techniques had the worst outcomes in terms of pain and fatigue. My theory on this result is that even though these patients had learned a technique to alleviate pain, they didn't want to take the responsibility for their own state of health. They were people who wanted a magic bullet.

When our center's practitioners offer treatments to new patients, they like to tailor sessions to each person's preferred method of learning—that is, visual, auditory, or by body movement. Each session runs about thirty minutes, usually started by focusing on one point. The trance is then deepened by counting breaths or imagining the experience of going down in an elevator or descending a staircase. When the patient reaches a deep enough state, the practitioner begins making positive suggestions to bring about certain physiological changes or goals. To return to full consciousness, the patient follows a reverse sequence—going up in the elevator or climbing the stairs.

All of this is done with the patient sitting in a comfortable chair or propped up in a hospital bed. We tape initial sessions and tell patients to play the tapes on a cassette player two times a day, once in the morning and once in the afternoon or evening. What we've discovered is that for some patients, such tapes become a daily or weekly activity months and even years after their surgery. Their self-hypnosis sessions, taped at a time when they were critically ill—some near death—are so deeply rooted in their minds as a path to relaxation that listening to the tapes invariably produces favorable changes in breathing, heart rate, blood pressure, and muscle tension. The practitioner's familiar messages function as triggers that return the patient back to a calming comfort zone.

Surgeries inevitably require that patients undergo many uncomfortable, even painful procedures. One kind of procedure in many surgeries is having to insert a catheter, or tube, into a patient in order to drain fluid, administer a drug, provide a conduit to insert a measuring or other device, or for some reason to provide access to an organ. Catheterization usually doesn't require general anesthesia, and in fact the patient must be conscious for many such procedures. So the less tense a patient is, the less discomfort he or she will feel. For just this purpose, self-hypnosis audiotapes have been tailor-made for patients about to undergo catheterization. One woman wrote the following note after her catheterization:

> The tape provided a wonderful feeling of relaxation that lasted nearly an hour—almost like having been drugged, yet without the drawbacks of drugs.
>
> It provided a feeling of being distant from the procedure going on—yet not out of control and not being drugged.
>
> The tape allowed me to separate myself from the procedure without being estranged from my own body.
>
> The use of the tape is also a way of conveying to me, in a concrete way, that I am not merely another body on the table but someone the medical staff really cares enough about to try making the procedure more comfortable. I responded by not tensing up and by putting myself in a "removed" frame of mind that distances myself from my own body.

Guided imagery is a similar auditory and visual approach to harnessing the mind's power in order to elicit physical responses. Instead of the straightforward, positive suggestions and instructions that are given during hypnosis sessions, practitioners in guided imagery have patients focus on mental images that can reduce stress and slow their heart rates, stimulate the immune system, and reduce pain. As part of the rapidly emerging field of mind-body medicine, this technique can be learned through the use of audiotapes, group participation, or private one-on-one sessions with a practitioner. Patients who take to such therapy, as with hypnosis, regularly use their guided imagery tapes long after they leave the hospital.

Whatever pathway to a mind-initiated state of relaxation is used by patients, the physical results are similar. Dr. Herbert Benson of the Mind/Body Medical Institute of New England Deaconess Hospital and Harvard Medical School popularized the term "relaxation response" in his book of the same title. He and his research colleagues have spent many years studying the effects and practical medical uses of this natural physical process, which can be viewed as the opposite of our adrenaline-pumping "fight-or-flight response." While this kind of reaction to a threat—physical or emotional, real or imagined—has helped us survive as a species in hostile or stressful situations, the long-term effects of the fight-or-flight response may lead to permanent, harmful physiological changes—particularly the cardiovascular kind we typically see in heart disease patients.

Research has shown that relaxation techniques used during surgery can affect degrees of consciousness in anesthetized patients. One landmark study, dubbed the "Robinson Crusoe" study, was carried out in South Africa in 1965. Fifty anesthetized patients who were undergoing surgery were briefly told Daniel Defoe's story of Crusoe's shipwreck. At the same time, fifty other randomly selected anesthetized patients underwent surgery, but these people had not been told the story of Robinson Crusoe and his friend, Friday. Later, when the patients from both groups woke up, they were asked, "Do you remember the operation?" They all answered no. Then they were asked, "Do you remember the pain?" They answered they did not. "Do you remember any stories being told?" Again, no. But then patients were asked one last question: "What does the word 'Friday' mean to you?" The people who did not hear the Crusoe story answered that Friday was the last day of the work week. However, of the patients who heard the story, about half answered, "Robinson Crusoe." Obviously, something had reached the minds of the supposedly deeply anesthetized patients.

Such a notion contradicts the popular image of patients under general anesthesia as zonked-out, corpselike bodies with no link to the conscious world, as pliable and mentally unresponsive as human-size rag dolls. To the surgical team, such an inert body has no personality and is simply a medical challenge, an object in need of attention. The "Crusoe" study and others have proven this view to be inaccurate. Open-heart-surgery patients, expecially, who receive anesthetics that minimally depress the heart's functioning and consequently are less likely to suppress the subconscious mind, may well be aware of what's going on during their surgery.

But can we quantify this awareness? When my research assistants and I studied the effects of music on anesthetized patients in the OR, I posed another question we might tackle: "Do relaxation tapes help patients get through surgery?" In order for us to come up with a practical, clinically useful answer, we had to divide the question into smaller ones: First, do people have the ability to hear while on the heart-lung bypass machine? Secondly, if so, can we condition this awareness? And thirdly, can we condition this awareness so that patients heal better faster?

With the parameters of our study defined, we began to record three levels of brain waves—early, middle, and late latency. Each wave corresponded to a different level of electrical activity in the brain or "awareness," with the middle one indicating at least subconscious cognition of external stimuli.

What happened when we put people to sleep and with a tape cassette played little click sounds in their ear? Before they went under anesthesia, they reacted to the clicks with strong, middle-latency period waves; after they were given gas and were unconscious, the middle waves continued to show patients were responding—there was awareness of the clicks. The response persisted when they were placed on the heart-lung machine and their hearts were stopped. Only in the cooling period could the patient eliminate this awareness. The answer to our question was obvious: every patient we examined could hear while under anesthesia.

Now, could we condition this awareness? Two of my research collaborators—neurologist Ron Emerson and anesthesiologist Dave Adams—with the help of our linguistics department, created two sets of word pairs. This was in itself a major accomplishment of the program—to have mainstream, accomplished researchers investigating complementary therapies in hard-science fashion. The word-pair sets were arranged from highest likelihood to lowest likelihood of a patient randomly guessing the correct correlating word. That is, if given "black" as the stimulus on an audiotape, 70 percent of respondents would answer "white," 20 percent would say "brown," and 10 percent would give miscellaneous answers. If, however, the patients heard "black-brown" as the correct word pair on the tape, would they now answer white or brown more frequently when prompted several days after the surgery. We found that patients would shift to the "brown" response when hearing the word "black," which demonstrates a change in implicit memory. The study showed that we *can* condition a person's awareness under anesthesia.

Everyone has an active subconscious when asleep. We dream and we think, and if somebody yells, "Fire!" we automatically know what to do, where our clothes are, what to grab, how to get out and get to safety. That's our subconscious guiding us. It's always aware, alert, protecting us. What we were doing with subliminal suggestions was attempting to tap the subconscious mind's ability to affect the body.

As for our third question—whether or not we can condition patients to heal better and faster—the jury is still out. One of our trials tested two groups of heart-disease patients, tape users and a control group of non-tape users. We wanted to see if such conditioning affected the incidence of atrial fibrillation—the rapid, erratic beating of the receiving chambers, or atria, of the heart. Treating the "afib" condition, which occurs in one of every three patients, is the single most expensive part of post-op care. But, if we could train patients to keep their blood pressure and heart rate normal, we would see if they can also avoid the afib problem and probably, in time, be able to answer a modified version of our original "big" question, "Can self-hypnosis and visualization therapy help patients get through surgery?"

One of the most popular auditory therapies is a set of six relaxation tapes, which patients listen to on headphones before, during, and after surgery. The words evoke various images—paradise-like beaches, rolling green hills, lush meadows, cool, quiet forests, and other serene natural environments—for the listener to envisage. The sound frequencies of the words, which are like musical tones, are known as "bineural beats." Two distinct sounds, or beats, are played—one in the right ear, the other in the left—which the brain then integrates into yet a third sound.

This integration of the left and right hemispheres of the brain is thought to help the body relax. Though we don't yet know exactly how they work, some patients who listen to these tapes claim to feel less stress than those who don't. The audiotape patients often have more stable blood pressure, lower heart rates and slower, deeper respiration. Many also require fewer pain and sleep medications after surgery.

But there's a certain suspension of disbelief that's required. For Joe Luciano, at first that was tough. His cardiologist had referred to him tersely as "a forty-five-year-old fella with new onset chest pain and significant three-vessel disease—needs open-heart surgery this week." Joe was a muscular, robust guy with thinning hair and an open, friendly face—but his eyes looked scared.

"I've never had to go to a hospital before," he said, "and I gotta tell you I'm a little antsy. But I got these blockages in my heart arteries, and I want them cleaned out."

I explained that for best results there had to be more to it than that. Joe wasn't just submitting himself as a patient with no more involvement than signing a consent form. But when I mentioned his emotional state and the various complementary therapies we had available, Joe gave a nervous chuckle. "Hold it, Doc," he said, "I just want to get my bum ticker fixed. I'm not a touchy-feely kind of person."

I named some of the more acceptable therapies—hypnotherapy, massage, and yoga—but all the while Joe was shaking his head. "Sorry," he insisted. "I don't think I'm going to be interested."

"Okay," I said. "There's no pressure. Just give these therapies a little more thought. So, tell me about the blockages. Where do you think they came from?"

"Smoking. I smoke a pack a day."

Joe confessed that while his wife prepared to drive him to the hospital, he had slipped a pack of cigarettes into his jacket. Even knowing that cigarettes could have contributed to his problem, he thought he might need a smoke to calm his nerves.

"I always thought," he added, "that if you go to the hospital, they'll find something wrong with you. If it turns out to be something big, I don't want to know about it."

Clearly Joe was convinced that surgery, our treatment plans—even quitting smoking—were painful things that would be imposed on or "done to" him. He felt like a passive follower of his doctors' whims rather than an active participant in the quest for health. "If I need surgery," he was saying, gazing out the window, "let's just get it over with."

Somehow I had to change Joe's attitude, and it struck me that the most effective approach might be to describe treatment as analogous to a process Joe already knew. I'd been told that Joe coached high school sports for twenty-five years, so I began: "Joe, before a big game, don't you want your players to be mentally ready?"

"Of course. You know, no distractions, keep your mind on the game."

"Exactly," I said. "Now, how do you do that?"

"I tell them to picture their favorite play—that all they've got to do is close their eyes and watch the perfect play, the way it's supposed to happen. That usually works."

"Well, think of me as your coach and you're on my surgical team. You're not a spectator, you're not the ball, you're not even just another player. You're a critical player—the quarterback or at least the blocking back. You're the key player and for you this really is a sudden-death game."

Joe nodded and cleared his throat.

"So you owe it to yourself and your team to prepare yourself for the game in every way you can," I went on. I asked him to meet with Jery Whitworth of the Complementary Care Center to get more of an overview of the various therapies and, later, with the individual practitioners, who would demonstrate their treatments—everything from reflexology to therapeutic touch—so he could pick out some to try. "Anything you don't feel comfortable with, you just tell us and we'll stop," I promised. "We're not going to force you to do anything."

"Fair enough," Joe said, still nervous but willing to listen.

When I dropped in later, Jery was just testing Joe's susceptibility to hypnotic suggestion. Induced successfully in a matter of minutes, Joe was an excellent candidate for hypnotherapy. Afterward, he blinked his eyes open, saying that he felt quite relaxed yet clear-eyed and not groggy as he'd be if he'd just awakened from a nap. So over the next two days Jery audiotaped several half-hour sessions that Joe could listen to over and over again to relieve his fear and anxiety. "You'll feel yourself sinking down into the bed," one tape begins, "you're going down, down, down . . ." As I'd hoped, Joe became addicted to the feeling of almost instant, restorative peace.

The night before surgery, I met with Joe again to praise him for rising to the challenge of working toward his own recovery. "You did the drills," I said, "you practiced what you have to do. Now you're ready for tomorrow's game. I'll get you through the first half and the third quarter. But in the fourth quarter you take over. The rest is going to be up to you."

Joe played his hypnosis tapes throughout the operation, which took three and a half hours, and when we wheeled him into the recovery room, he still had the tape running on auto-reverse. Over the next two hours he regained consciousness without a hitch, and within a day was ready to leave the ICU. He had calmed himself so well through self-hypnosis that he kept his heart rate and blood pressure normal, with no additional heart medications, and he didn't need morphine to manage his pain. Most patients undergoing such radical operations need a breathing tube for twelve to eighteen hours after surgery, but Joe's came out almost immediately. Just four days later, he was able to go home.

What happened? How could someone recover so fast after having his chest cleaved open?

Joe's mental preparation made all the difference. In the forty-eight hours between admission and surgery, he had shifted from an acted-upon receiver to a determined doer—and he came out a winner. His steadfast approach to one of life's biggest challenges—fighting disease—calls to mind the approach taken by Psyche, in the Greek myth, to view her mysterious lover, Cupid. The god of Love, Cupid became enamored of Psyche, a beautiful princess, and swept her away to an isolated castle where he'd make love to her in darkness and leave by daybreak because mortals were forbidden to look at gods. But Psyche couldn't resist the temptation to see her lover, and so one night as he slept, she came to him bearing a knife and a lighted lamp.

Why both? As Dr. Jean Bolen says, Psyche needed to become enlightened to face the unknown, but she also needed to be armed to deal with the consequences. Metaphorically, Joe had embraced the knife of surgery, but he also needed a lamp—the enlightenment to face his disease. He needed both conventional or "allopathic" and complementary medicines.

Coach Joe Luciano, whose physical and emotional recovery rose to the top of my success-story list, still listens to his tapes when he gets anxious, such as before games and dental visits. "We had a lot of overtime games this season," he told me. "I could feel my heart race thumpety-thump, but I was fine, just like normal."

"How's the stress management?" I asked.

"Whenever a tough situation comes at me," he said, "I just tell myself that I've got this imaginary shield—a big plastic imaginary shield—that I put up around me. I suck in a few deep breaths, take a minute to gather my thoughts, and then I deal with the situation."

"How about the urge to smoke?"

"Doc, that pack of cigarettes I took with me to the hospital— I put it in a kitchen drawer. That's where it's going to stay. That's me as I was. It's my reminder that now I live right."

Jerry Boyko's case was more dire, for his heart was beyond repair. The tall, handsome, successful importer of steel products had to wait nearly two months for a transplant while an LVAD kept him alive.

Early on, when I informed him of the complementary therapies we had available, he raised his eyebrows. Like Joe Luciano, he was a doubter, who lumped all such healing approaches into a vague pie-in-the-sky camp. But Jerry Boyko had an unusually aggressive, cooperative attitude toward participation in his own treatment, surgery, and recovery. "If a relative were having this operation," he asked me, "would you make sure he or she used complementary medicine?"

"Absolutely," I replied.

"Fine," he said without hesitating. "I'll try it."

His first enthusiasm was for yoga stretches, but he soon began to prefer his self-hypnosis tapes—that is, recordings of his sessions with a hypnotherapist. Boyko told me the tapes helped him cope with the fears and anxiety he felt about the entire hospitalization process. Besides the fact he was completely dependent on a mechanical pump thumping inside him day and night, the taped messages also allowed him some confidence in looking toward a successful transplant. The instructions to coach him just prior and during surgery were mostly to get him to relax. But the post-op suggestions that were part of the taped session were so that he would bleed little, heal quickly, and need only a minimal amount of pain medication. He never saw the upcoming surgery as an ordeal but as a challenge that would save his life.

By the time we informed him that we had a possible donor heart for him, he and his wife, Leslie, were thoroughly prepared.

It was 1:40 in the morning when we found out that we had a car-accident victim who was a good match to provide him a new heart. While Boyko was readying himself mentally, our anesthesiologists began preparing him for the transplant surgery. By 2:45, Boyko was stretched out on the OR table, unconscious, breathing through a respirator, his headphones on his ears. Throughout the entire operation his auto-reverse Walkman would feed him soothing music and word images to keep him relaxed. Just after three, I began the surgery.

As delicately as I could, I opened the chest bone from top to bottom with an electric saw. As I prepared the way for removing his diseased, flaccid, battered-looking heart, he was relaxing, blocking out any subconscious anxiety. I glanced over the draped surgical area to peek at his earphones and cassette player just to make sure the tape was still playing and the headphones were on his ears. The Walkman was fine.

His heart had many more adhesions than I expected, and during the dissection I created a hole in his right ventricle. In just about every open-heart operation there is a time when, if you make the wrong decision, you'll kill the patient. In Boyko's surgery that time had arrived. I had two choices: I could pull on the heart and risk ripping the hole bigger and very possibly killing him, or I could wait and retreat, covering the chest for a while and keeping his blood loss small while I quickly put a catheter in his groin to connect him to the bypass machine. Experience told me I should go with the second option, which we call "crashing on bypass." I did the procedure and Boyko remained unaffected. For now his mind was in a safe zone, keeping him centered.

While he was on the bypass machine, I used an electrical burning device to slice away the stubborn tissue encasing the front of the heart. Slowly and meticulously I worked my way forward, looking for clues to where I was. It was like doing a jigsaw puzzle. I'd see a piece over here and another over there, and I'd know what was in between. But I had to cut down these targets without injuring vital structures hidden within the scar. Finally I "unstuck" the heart, overcoming what could have been a disastrous setback in the whole procedure. I was entering the same centered place that my patient had been inhabiting for the past three hours.

It was almost five in the morning when the organ harvesters entered with the heart in its Igloo cooler. Before I even opened the lid, I asked for music for the OR team. The anesthesiologist put a CD of Vivaldi flute concertos into the player—"Good-morning music," she called it. After I took the diseased heart out of the chest cavity, I lifted the pink, vibrant donor heart out of the cooler and examined the muscle surface and severed mouths of its various openings. Finally, I started the painstaking job of connecting the atria, aorta, and pulmonary arteries to Boyko's corresponding vessels. Unlike other unprepared patients whom energy healers have described as "spiritually jumping up to the roof" and running around crazily, Boyko remained calm and within his body.

Around six-thirty, I was about to take him off the bypass machine and watch the most exciting part of a transplant—when the new heart starts to beat and life returns to a patient. We injected blood into the dormant organ, waited for about forty-five seconds, then gently slapped the heart with two fingers—a little kick start to wake it up. We waited. Suddenly the muscle sprang to life, then the new heartbeat settled into a steady, strong rhythm.

At 7:12 A.M., after I gave the order to go off the bypass machine, Boyko began to pump blood on his own, and I stepped back from the table to stretch. I checked his relaxation tape. It was still revolving on auto-reverse. He was calmly aware of his body's return to normal circulation, and hours later, the first thing Boyko requested when he regained consciousness were his tapes. He was determined to be on the quick track to recovery.

As it turned out, he mended faster than most patients, and he used little more than Tylenol for pain. I asked him the same question he had used to start our discussion of the potential benefits of complementary medicine months earlier: "If a relative were having this operation, would you make sure he used complementary medicine?" Jerry Boyko just cocked his head, gave me a wink, and smiled.

5

Rainbow Man

Music heard so deeply
that it is not heard at all,
but you are the music
while the music lasts.

—T. S. Eliot

Since I was a kid growing up spending summers with my parents in Turkey, I've been enthralled by the Bosporus, the strait separating Asia and Europe. I liked walking along the crowded shoreline road near the Bosporus Bridge, smelling fish and fruits, listening to the cries of vendor and seagulls, or just gazing at that rippling expanse of blue water that is the meeting point of East and West. For centuries armies battled over the Bosporus, and each new invader made its mark. Byzantium became the Christian Constantinople, which was conquered in 1453 by an Ottoman, Mehmet the Conqueror, who claimed it for Islam and renamed it Istanbul. Since the Muslim Turks were not destructive people, they built on the richness of the city, which prospered even as Europe was mired in the Dark Ages. It became the trading post where Europe and Asia met, one of the great crossroads of the world. Even now, Istanbul remains an often enigmatic place where different cultures, different ways of thinking, can unite and be reconciled, even fused.

Recently I returned to Istanbul to give a lecture on new

advances in heart surgery. Late one afternoon I slipped out of my parents' waterfront villa, their Turkish home, and walked along that same busy stretch of shoreline road. I thought again of those Muslim Turks, remembering that they would hire Christians and Jews to translate ancient Greek writings on health and treating disease; and so while medicine stagnated in Europe for a millennium, the Islamic world made major breakthroughs by building on the lost traditions. Looking up at the Bosporus Bridge, I thought of the George Washington Bridge, visible from my window in the cardiac-surgery intensive-care unit at Columbia Presbyterian in New York. I had battled for the lives of many patients in that ICU and knew that Western medicine had lots of answers—of this I was proud. But often we didn't have enough of the answers, and I mused that perhaps my Eastern roots would show me some new questions to ask.

That very night my parents had invited some friends and relatives to hear a musician who was said to heal with music. This healer-scholar, a man with a doctorate in philosophy who worked as a psychologist, had scoured Central Asia, from eastern Turkey to Mongolia, in search of information about the ancient tonal-healing arts and had published numerous articles about how and why it worked. He had even made his own versions of traditional instruments.

I hadn't previously used music as a treatment for specific ailments, but of course, I was intrigued. I had heard that many centuries ago folk healers among the nomads in eastern Turkey and Central Asia used different tones to "cure" the sick, and I also knew that soothing music or calming sounds could lower a person's blood pressure, heart rate, and levels of stress hormones, as well as stimulate the release of pleasure-producing endorphins. But I wasn't so sure such effects actually healed or aided healing.

Just after sunset, a little man with a twisted spine stepped into the living room with an armload of various stringed instruments. Rahmi Oruc Guvenc (pronounced O-*ruch* Gu-*vench*) was well under five feet tall, middle-aged, and remarkably handsome in a jaunty black beret and a folksy embroidered shirt. A younger man and a heavyset barefoot woman in a long peasant dress followed him, carrying various flutes, drums, wooden instruments, and a large copper basin.

We gathered around in a semi-circle as Rahmi carefully removed a chamois covering from what looked like a big, pear-shaped lute with three strings. He began to strum the big lute-like *oud* propped on his lap, singing a soft Turkish folk melody in a rich tenor voice. Beside him the young woman, a cup in each hand, poured water into the copper basin, creating the soothing sound of a fountain. As the rhythm and singing picked up in pace, the tall man rose and started to dance, turning round and round, slowly waving his arms up and down. Guvenc revved up the song to a frenzied pitch, goading the dancer to spin faster and faster and the water to run quicker.

The young man reminded me of Turkey's religious Sufi dancers, the dervishes who whirl themselves into trancelike states. I had seen them as a child in Konya, my father's hometown and center of Sufi activities in the world for many centuries. The dancers, spinning at about sixty revolutions per minute, pray and meditate while listening to the soothing, repetitious music. Legend has it that the whirling began in 1247, when a spiritual leader named Jalaluddin Rumi, or Mevlana ("our master"), began to spin on an axis of agony and rapture until his heart was pure. As he whirled he uttered a series of spontaneous prayers for a friend and spiritual teacher who had been murdered by Mevlana's jealous followers. His prayerful utterings eventually became the seed for a long poem that's revered alongside the Koran as a sacred text.

One poetic piece of Mevlana's wisdom describes the symbolic power of the music Guvenc played for us that night. A man, Mevlana said, is like a reed, cut away and turned into a flute. Like the reed, he finds that his life, lived far from its source, turns empty and hollow. The pain and wonder of this realization pierces holes in his heart. As the wind blows through the flute, it wails with its broken heart. It is pain that becomes music, the music of a yearning life being lived. As I listened to the music and watched the whirling dancer, I could easily imagine the yearning sound of a flute.

Gradually, the tempo eased up, then slowed; the dancer began to sway, and the water pouring grew louder. They were done. After a moment of silence, Guvenc asked how we felt. Like many others, I felt relaxed, clear-headed. Some of my relatives singled out their necks as being much more relaxed. The handsome little genie at the end of the room smiled. "The pieces I play," he said in Turkish, "are meant to soothe different parts of the body. What you just heard was for the neck."

He explained that sounds based on a five-tone scale affect the limbic system of the brain, and emotional changes in listeners can be detected on an EEG, a test that measures brain waves. In this way, he pointed out, music therapy has helped in the treatment of autistic children and certain types of pain, cramps, and muscular spasms usually treated by physical therapy.

Guvenc left me feeling as though I had imbibed a mind-altering substance, and I started to imagine how certain patients of mine would respond to his music. Some had complained that before they were anesthetized in the operating room, they could hear the nurses discussing their afternoon duties or the heart-lung machine perfusionist describing a play at a Yankees game—making them feel depersonalized, as an inanimate object on which a job had to be done. They had difficulty focusing their healing energies because the people around them were on a different wavelength. Music, I realized, could block out such distractions and, perhaps, as Guvenc maintains, offer additional therapeutic benefits.

I asked Guvenc for some tapes, and he later sent me more than a dozen, with music designed to treat various parts of the body and specific ailments. But in Western, or allopathic, medicine, we don't recognize many of the disease categories his music aimed to treat. There were tapes for lethargy, tapes for circulation, tapes for "energy patterns"—all new and different diagnostic categories. So my first task would be to translate these foreign paradigms of health and disease into terms that my professional brethren and, even more important, my patients could understand. I would have to link the traditional medicine of the East, where my cultural roots were, with the science of the West, which I was trained to practice.

Not long after I returned from Turkey, I got a fax from my cardiologist colleague Howard Levin about a critically ill fifty-seven-year-old black male named Johnny Copeland who was "going down the tubes"—his lame heart was about to fail him. "He gets an LVAD or he dies," Howard said bluntly.

I arrived at the hospital about 9:45 that evening and went to the waiting room to meet Copeland's anxious family, his wife, Sandra and his teenage son and daughter. Mrs. Copeland seemed surprised that I wasn't a much older physician. We shook hands and talked about operating on her husband. "Ohhh-kay," she said in a drawl, eyebrows raised, "But aren't you tired?"

"No, I'm fine," I said. "I'm used to doing this. But I think the three of you should go home. For the next six hours your husband will be mine, and you won't be able to do anything for him. Save your energy, so you can help him get better when he wakes up."

"You sure about that?" she said. Like loved ones of most patients in similar circumstances, she did not want to leave. But eventually she agreed.

The surgical team had already wheeled Copeland into an operating room, and had him prepped, anesthetized and waiting for me as I scrubbed for surgery. The cardiac operating-room suites form their own unique core, with large glass panes to allow surgeons scrubbing at the aluminum sinks outside to observe the patient being prepped and watch for signs of trouble. Inside I could see the perfusionists, who run the heart-lung machine that enables us to stop the heart, meticulously cleaning their metal and plastic pumps and preparing the tubing that I would eventually insert into the heart. The OR suites, each the size of a small conference hall, house three tables of fine surgical instruments, sutures, and other devices, which two OR nurses keep groomed and counted like hens guarding their eggs.

The operation started out smoothly. I sliced the skin over the sternum in a long, even line, pulling back the skin and muscle, sawing through the chest bone, spreading open the chest with a foot-long metal retractor, cauterizing the tiny bleeders—the vessels I had severed—and exposing the heart organ. There, pulsing beneath a thin sac of tissue called the pericardium, I got a first glimpse of my target. As I opened the sac, I saw the fist-size heart wriggling like a fish caught on a line. I connected it to the heart-lung machine and plugged in the LVAD.

Then complications set in—the pressure in Johnny's lungs was very high, which impeded blood flow even with a well-working LVAD. As his blood pressure dropped, we added one drug, then another, and a third—all with limited success. Finally, with an intricate concoction of medications, we got Johnny stabilized and rolled him off to an intensive care recovery room. The operation had taken nearly five hours.

Heart surgeons call the time immediately after an operation the bewitching hour because that's when big problems, if there will be any, occur. In Johnny Copeland's case, I wasn't at all satisfied that he was out of danger, so I decided to stay near and sleep in my office. After calling Sandra to report that her husband was now resting with his new heart pump, I rolled out my sleeping bag on my cushion-covered bench by the window and instantly fell asleep.

About an hour later, the phone ringing woke me up. "Dr. Oz," a nurse said with some urgency, "Copeland's blood pressure just dropped to nothing. He's arresting! Come quickly!"

I raced to the ICU, where a nurse was already doing chest compressions, in order to keep some blood flowing to Johnny's brain. I did a quick check, then gave Johnny some very strong drugs to see if they could raise his blood pressure, which they did, but just barely.

"Let's get him to the OR!" I shouted. We disconnected lines and tubes, yanked the bed out, swung it around, and propelled our nearly lifeless patient out of the ICU and down the hallway. Two nurses scampered alongside, holding up plastic tubes and IV bags. But who would help me with the surgery? It was nearly five o'clock in the morning, and my team had gone home.

I got lucky. As we careened around a corner, I spotted Robbie Ashton, the young resident who had coordinated our hypnosis tests and who, coincidentally, was on a transplant team scheduled to operate early that morning. He just happened to be going out to "harvest" the donated heart that was being delivered to the hospital.

"Robbie!" I yelled. "I need you. Grab the bed! We're going to open this guy."

We shoved the bed through the double doors of the OR, but by then Johnny's eyes had rolled back eerily in their sockets so that only the whites showed. For a split second I thought we had lost him. No blood pressure.

"Knife!" I shouted. The borrowed surgical team moved into position. With one swipe I cut through three layers of Johnny's recently closed chest. "Wire cutters!" Quickly, I snipped out the six wires that held the sternum together. The heart lay lifeless beneath the bone—distended, blue, swollen. I wormed one hand into the cavity and began to squeeze it, trying to mimic normal contractions. Slowly, his blood pressure returned, although the blips on the monitor were barely visible. I asked Robbie to take over the hand compressions. "Keep the blood moving to his head," I ordered. Although the blood pressure was low, if I could keep his brain alive for another few minutes, I could reinsert tubes from the heart-lung machine and restore a safe blood pressure, if only for a short while. I stabbed the aorta and right atrium with a stiletto blade, then quickly inserted the bypass tubes. Blood whooshed through the transparent plastic tubes;

Johnny was back on the heart-lung machine. The gambit had worked—so far.

About twenty minutes had passed from the time I got the phone call to the moment we connected him. Before his heart stopped beating, his blood pressure remained below an absurdly low 30. Then the pressure started rising—first 35, then 45, 65, finally up around a safer 80. In the OR, the regular *bip-bips* of the oxymeter machine say two things: how fast the patient's heart is beating and how much oxygen is in the blood. The higher the tone, the higher the oxygen; the lower the tone, the lower the oxygen. Johnny's rhythmic, tone-rising oxymeter *bips* were like fine music. Steady, strong.

But were we too late? I tried to figure out why he'd gone sour on us. I tinkered with a few of his medications, then adjusted the ventilator and finally optimized the LVAD settings. But the most important treatment was tincture of time. I decided to take him off the heart-lung machine by putting a temporary plastic pump in him, which would help push the blood across the lungs. This pump did the work of the right side of the heart. With the LVAD pumping for the left side, Johnny would have both ventricles supported—one right, one left. So I put the second pump in— it's a bigger, longer contraption that actually remains connected outside the body. Then I spent hours more trying to stop his bleeding—a result of the trauma of bringing him back from the edge.

"What do you think?" Robbie asked as we wheeled our battered patient out of the OR to a recovery room.

I couldn't answer for a moment. Not so much from fatigue but from a sense of profound disappointment. "He could be brain dead," I said. We both knew you couldn't really tell for sure until we got the heart—bolstered by the two pumps—to work properly.

In the ICU, Sandra and her children looked petrified. I told them I had done the best I could and that we had operated on many similar patients who had done well, although Johnny's case had been complicated. Sandra asked if there was anything they could do. "Pray," I said. "That's the best thing you can do. And stay by his bedside. Let him know you're there and you care."

I went home to my apartment across the Hudson late that night and slept for the first time in two days. I kept dreaming Johnny had awakened, but when I called at six a.m., the evening-shift nurse said, "No movements, not yet."

On the trip back to the hospital, I kept tapping the Seek button on the car radio. Suddenly, I heard a familiar name. "That's Johnny Copeland!" the voice said. "Next we're going to hear 'The Rainbow Song.' " Was the word out about Johnny's hospitalization? Or was it a coincidence they were playing his material that morning? In all the time laboring over this man, I hadn't even known he was a celebrated blues singer known as the Texas Twister.

When I got to the ICU, I could tell by the glum expressions of the family and the nursing staff that Johnny was still profoundly unconscious. With a breathing tube in his mouth, tubes running out of his chest, and monitor lines running to various parts of his body, he looked like a pathetic, dormant puppet.

I put an arm around Sandra's shoulder. "I think his heart's going to recover," I said, "so let's be innovative in trying to awaken him." I told her about hearing his song on the radio and asked her if she had any tapes of his music.

"Yeah, he loves his music," Sandra said, and fished a tape out of her purse. I stuck it in a Walkman and placed the headphones over his ears. Guvenc, the hunchbacked music therapist, had been emphatic that music can reach deeply into the brain, well below our conscious mind. If Johnny could be reached this way, maybe with therapy he could be stimulated back to full consciousness.

I left the room to do rounds among other patients. For some reason—a premonition maybe—I came back about ten minutes later. I checked the monitors. Johnny's vital indicators, bleeped out in graph lines and numbers on the various screens, were the same as when I had left him. Then I looked at the Walkman to see if the tape was still going and the volume was okay. As I leaned over the bed, my face coming close to his, I noticed Johnny was crying. Little tears were welling from under his eyelids. In seconds the tears were dropping off his cheeks. "He's alive!" I exclaimed, suddenly excited. "He's not brain dead!"

I explained to the team and to Johnny's family that since he could still respond emotionally to the music, he hadn't lost cognitive function. For a long, heavy moment Sandra, who was seated by the foot of the bed, was silent. Then she smiled, stood up, and wiped her husband's face. For a long time she held his hand, squeezing it every now and then, tears on her own face.

Over the next seven days Johnny gradually came to. The headphones would stay on for hours, and he started moving his fingers and tapping his toes on the bed rail. His own music reached a part of him that technology could not. Like Sufi mystic dancers who elevate themselves to a higher level of existence through music and their spinning dance, Johnny was able to tap into a higher or more spiritual self. When Johnny's own blues first penetrated through the headset and vibrated the tympanic membrane, activating the auditory system and stimulating the correct neural synapse, he was recognizing the tones—he was living in the now. He wasn't worried about yesterday or tomorrow, and fortunately he wasn't depressed by having to live at the mercy of a machine pumping his blood. He was happy while listening. In a very real way, Johnny was listening to the language of the heart, focusing his efforts on recovery.

But I didn't know if he would ever play his guitar and sing again. What if I'd given him his body back but not his life, his music? It happens all the time that we operate on people, they go through hell and back, and they survive, but they don't come "back to life." They can never return to their previous careers or daily routines. Their memories may fail or they may no longer be able to reason logically. The person entrusted to us before the operation is gone. What happens then?

But when he was able to speak again, Johnny told me, "The blues is still the same." He put his hand on his chest. "The feeling is still in here." He had only one serious complaint. "Doc, I can't compose."

I figured he might be having emotional problems adjusting to his slowed-down pace and his restriction to staying within six hours' travel time of the hospital, in case a matchable heart became available to replace his present pump-aided organ. But Johnny explained that what kept him from writing was the incessant whooshing, *ker-plunking* sound of the LVAD. "I used to compose late at night when everything was quiet," he said. "I could forget myself. But this gadget here won't let me forget. Throws off my timing." He shrugged and added that at least he could still play his old songs and he was putting a lot more emotion into them.

Five months later, after a slow but steady recovery, Johnny had his first public gig since coming back from the dead. The marquee over Manny's Car Wash, a blues bar on Manhattan's Upper East Side, touted the Texas Twister's return in big red letters: WELCOME BACK. It seemed like half the hospital staff showed up, certainly most of the ICU nurses and cardiothoracic staff. Nurses, doctors, residents, students, physician's assistants, orderlies, janitors, even people from the business offices and many of our other LVAD patients—all crammed themselves into the rear area near the small corner stage. These people had bathed him, fed him, transfused him. They knew him intimately, knew the best and the worst of his vital signs. I had opened him up and held his heart in my hands. In a clinical and emotional sense, we were more than caretakers. We were family.

When Johnny emerged from backstage, the shrieks and howls were deafening. He waved and grinned, then sat down with his guitar and adjusted the mike on its gooseneck stand. As he hit the strings with a swipe of his hand, his five backup musicians erupted into hard-driving Texas-style blues. At one point Johnny threw his head back and I saw the whites of his eyes, just as I had seen them on the OR table as his blood pressure plummeted. That had been a petrifying moment, watching death sneak into my patient, but now as his eyes rolled back, he was celebrating the gift of survival with his soul-felt music.

About an hour later, Johnny Clyde Copeland finished his set with "Life's Rainbow," his signature song. Whoever heard it that night, especially us up front, connected with the words about a person's love shining like a rainbow. Again, he surveyed his friends, then cleared his throat, nodded to our table, and said, "This one's for you, Dr. Oz. You're my wizard."

The beat was slow, harmonica and electric guitar blending in a long, plaintive cry. Then Johnny eased in with, "Everybody say yeah . . . say yeah!" We did, then he sang on with a deep, soulful edge:

> . . . I went and stood on the mountain,
> and I had a little talk with the sky.
> And it showed me a beautiful rainbow.
> And it said, Johnny, that represents life.
> Love's got to shine like a rainbow for everyone to see
> and at the end of the rainbow—you're your pot of gold.

That evening with Johnny for me was a culmination of my growing conviction that music could aid in the healing process. This belief began when Guvenc, the Turkish music therapist and researcher, enlightened me on the ancient techniques of what we now call music therapy. If our hearts provide us with the pulse of life, then music connects us in a direct way with our own natural rhythmical instrument—the body. Certain sounds, certain tones, can measurably decrease physical signs of stress and worry, such as a rapid heart rate, quick, shallow breathing, and the release of adrenaline into the bloodstream. Whether we listen to blues, Bach, or the simplest lullaby, our bodies are capable of reacting by relaxing, by tapping into the subconscious mind. In Johnny Copeland's case, his own music became his best ally from the world of complementary healing.

❧ 6 ❧

Lessons from Wat Po

The way to health is a scented bath
and an oiled massage every day.

—Hippocrates

Almost all the patients entering our medical center are eager to try massage. Some feel it's the most relaxing of all the complementary medicine therapies we offer, but of course, it offers more benefits than just unkinking the knots and soothing the muscles. In some cultures and countries, therapeutic massage has been for centuries a mainstay in protecting and promoting health. In Thailand, for instance, massage is an integral part of their traditional healing system. While on a visit there I discovered firsthand some of the practical and even religious side of this ancient, most basic remedy for all kinds of ailments, from muscular pain to supposedly irreversible paralysis.

My wife, Lisa, and I had just rented horses to ride on the beach, but I could barely get mine to move. He looked strong and was supposed to be faster than Lisa's mount, but he was stubborn and indifferent to all my whistles, shouts, heel kicks, and slaps on his haunches. So I poked along to the end of the beach, where Lisa was waiting, and we turned the horses around to head back.

That's when my stallion decided to bolt. He took off like a thoroughbred exploding out of the gate. I hung on, trying to rein him in, slow him down. No way—he was in full gallop. All kinds of people—kids, families—were on the beach, so we went dodging in and out of the human traffic. Rather than panic and jump off, I grabbed his mane and held on for dear life.

By the time the horse stopped, I was battered and sore from the unwanted thrill ride. As I limped away, a small, wiry, older woman approached and offered to give me a massage. I plopped down on the warm sand, and my agile masseuse went to work on me, using every sharp angle on her body—elbows, knuckles, fingertips, knees, and feet. Her touch was deep as well as gentle. She pushed and pressed and kneaded my muscles, twisting me like a human pretzel, pulling this way, pushing that way, probing and gouging. Later, I learned that what she had given me was a traditional Thai body tonic massage, which the Thais use often to maintain their quality of life.

A few days later Lisa and I wandered down a crowded Bangkok side street and found an herbal clinic where "royal" Thai massage is practiced for healing purposes. Thais basically use two systems of medicine that are not mutually exclusive but often used in tandem, depending on whether the problem is chronic or acute. The Western-based system is, of course, practiced in modern hospitals and clinics, while the traditional form, steeped in Buddhist beliefs, relies on extensive herbal pharmacies, herbal steam baths, yoga, and the therapeutic massage that had been developed ages ago for royalty. Because commoners were not supposed to touch royalty, what developed was a two-finger method of deep massage on acupressure points that alleviate energy blockages along meridian paths familiar in Chinese and Indian traditions. Traditional Thai medicine is actually a bit of both and has a unique pharmacopoeia.

Out of curiosity I visited a large herbal pharmacy, which turned out to be a wonderfully fragrant emporium of thousands of different natural remedies for all kinds of chronic, mostly mi-

nor, ailments. On the main floor, crowded and busy with customers, neatly ordered mounds of bags, boxes, and sacks of ingredients filled the middle area. At one side counters were topped
by rows of wide-mouthed, covered jars of other items; on another side, more storage of boxed and bagged goods; and at the
far end were the scales, chopping blocks, and clerks. The recipes,
or prescriptions, had been handed down through generations, all
originally brought by monks from India and China, with many of
the arcane mixtures written originally in Sanskrit and Bali.
What struck me most was how much time and effort patients
must commit to their own treatments. It's not like taking pills—
they must prepare each remedy in elaborate procedures that
sometimes take hours in grinding, mixing, and cooking. Taking
care of their bodies is serious business—again, something Buddhism encourages.

At the herbal clinic I saw a one-year-old girl brought in by
her father. Her right arm hung at her side, paralyzed since birth.
Apparently the hospital doctor who delivered her resolved a
sure-death situation in a very difficult birth, but in pulling her,
he slipped a finger around her delicate little armpit, inadvertently tearing the nerve cluster that controls her arm.

In the West we have no satisfactory treatment for such an injury. It's an unfortunate, usually irreversible paralysis. But here
they were about to start a series of about two dozen therapeutic
massage treatments. First, one clinician examined the girl and
made a diagnosis. Then someone else took over and began the
pressure-point massage, stroking down on the arm patiently, over
and over. I discussed the probable results with a clinic healer and
was told that the likelihood of a cure wasn't high, but that in the
past they'd had some success in restoring movement to such affected arms.

While at the clinic I also learned that different yoga
stretches, breathing techniques, and positions are used for medicinal purposes. Originally the poses were taken from different
animal postures—like the down-dog and cobra poses. On the

grounds around some of the temples, or *wats*, I saw ancient stat-
ues of persons in various therapeutic positions, such as a squat-
ting posture that's recommended for strengthening hearts. And
on centuries-old walls I examined painted illustrations of human
figures with superimposed "maps" of energy pathways, or meridians, and acupressure points.

Acupressure, like its sister technique, acupuncture, has been
used in China and other parts of Asia for thousands of years to
relieve pain and improve organ function. Thought to be the
older of the two energy-healing systems, acupressure probably
was born with the natural human instinct to respond to a place
on the body that is injured, painful, or tense. Whereas acupuncture employs heated needles to puncture the skin and reach specific meridian points throughout the body, acupressure calls for
the firm force of hands, fingers, knuckles, and even feet to reach
the same pressure points. As with most techniques in the traditional, Eastern-based healing system, the goal is to bring a
balance, or harmony, in the body's flow of *chi*, or vital force.

Acupressure is especially effective in the relief of tension-
related ailments. In this healing system, tension is regarded as a
stagnation of bodily energies that flow through the nerves, lymphatics, blood vessels, and meridians. Finger pressure at specific
sites, for example, helps open up clogged channels, or energy
pathways, freeing blocked energy and relieving tension.

Before leaving Thailand, I had one last massage session, this
time an herbal massage given at a well-known temple called Wat
Po, where some of the country's best practitioners are trained.
The large room was crowded with customers lying on floor mats.
I was shown to a spot, and in minutes someone was pressing into
my bare back a small bag filled with various steamy, boiled herbs,
including casimar, camphor, borneal camphor, kiffer lime, lemon
grass, turmeric, and acacia. The little bag was hot but not painful
because the practitioner moved it very quickly from spot to spot.
When the massage ended, I was absolutely relaxed, my mind
calm but focused and alert.

As with so many healing approaches that Western medicine considers unconventional, massage has its roots in antiquity. Most ancient cultures practiced some form of healing by touching or rubbing, with shamans, priests, and folk healers performing the rituals used for relief of aches, pain, and soreness. In the tomb of the Egyptian physician Ankh-mahor, dated from around 2200 B.C., a bas-relief depicts a priest rubbing the foot of a seated man. Massage as a healing art was first mentioned in writing about three thousand years ago, first in China, then in ancient Persian medicinal descriptions and Indian texts on herbal medicine. Of course, we know from written references that ancient Greeks and Romans frequently used oil and herb massages. In the fourth century B.C., the Greek physician Hippocrates, considered the father of modern medicine, repeatedly extolled the curative and restorative qualities of massage.

In the West, massage was kept alive as a common folk practice especially among the Slavs, Finns, and Swedes. Elsewhere in the world—in India, China, Japan, the Americas, and some of the South Pacific Islands—various forms of massage developed and flourished as weapons against pain and illness. In Turkey, my own ancestral home, the so-called Turkish baths have flourished as a blend of ancient indigenous and Greco-Roman practices, which include much bathing, scrubbing, soapy washing, rinsing and plenty of vigorous massage while lying on marble platforms. Today, in the United States massage practitioners go through rigorous training, followed by thorough certification procedures. It is estimated that about 85,000 practitioners each year give 60 million treatments to 25 million Americans.

Besides the Chinese-derived acupressure and a similar technique in Japan called shiatsu, other popular kinds of massage include Swedish, deep-tissue, trigger-point (or neuromuscular), and sports massage. Generally, these treatments can be said to help the venous return of blood to the heart, stimulate lymph movement out of affected tissues, stretch such soft and connective tissue as skin, muscles, tendons, and ligaments, and affect the function of the stomach, small intestine, and colon. Massage can also help free endorphins, the pain-killing chemicals produced in the brain in response to stroking, kneading, stretching, and other movements of a massage therapist. Even a simple touch of a hand on the skin can lower blood pressure and heart rate.

Researchers at the University of Miami, Duke, and Harvard and investigators at Miami's Touch Research Institute have demonstrated in scores of controlled studies the beneficial results of massage on patients with a wide range of problems, from asthma and anxiety to migraines and diabetes. One study, for example, showed that prematurely born babies who are massaged three times a day for ten days are likely to be more alert, active, and responsive, and will gain weight 47 percent faster than non-massaged preemies. Explaining that neither group of babies drank more formula than the other, the study concluded the weight gain of the massaged babies was due to more efficient food absorption.

Massage has also been shown to have profound effects on the hormonal and immunologic systems. For example, rats undergoing belly massage will release oxytocin, an important hormone from the brain. In addition, AIDs patients will elevate their natural killer cells in the immune system after several massage sessions. Whether this change will help patients is unclear, but these findings point to a potential immunologic effect of massage.

My patients, especially those with mechanical heart pumps who were hospitalized for long periods of time, gave me a unique chance to study the beneficial effects of massage therapy. I was particularly interested in observing the movement of lymphatics, which function as a sort of trash-disposal system for our bodies. I had spent many years at the dinner table with my heart surgeon father-in-law, Gerald Lemole, discussing his early ideas on lymphatics and their role in atherosclerosis. Interestingly, music conductors, who are always moving their arms up and down and self-massaging their lymphatics, appear to have less atherosclerosis than people of similar age in other occupations. Lemole believed this narrowing, or "hardening," of the arteries was especially prevalent among heart-transplant patients because the lymphatic system doesn't regenerate in the new hearts, which can promote the buildup of fatty deposits in the arteries.

Our program offered a unique opportunity to study the effects of lymphatic massage, since sensors in the LVAD show us exactly how much blood is pumped out to a patient's tissues at all times. All the fluid in the body's veins and arteries passes through the lymphatic system, where waste products are removed. But then how does the lymphatic system get rid of the waste? Exercise can dramatically increase lymphatic drainage (and possibly improve the functioning of the body's immune system), but investigators have shown that when the foot pads of dogs are massaged, this stimulation has a similar effect. If we massaged the feet of our LVAD patients, recording their blood flow and lymphatic activity, would they get the same lymphatic drainage benefit? One very difficult case made a believer out of me.

Kory Boglarski, only sixteen years old, was the youngest patient in whom I had ever inserted an implantable LVAD. In fact, he was the youngest in the world ever to go home with an LVAD. When I first saw Kory with Jack and Peg, his parents, I was struck by his blond hair and blue eyes. He was a snow-board instructor in Connecticut, and even though it was the end of winter, he regretted missing the remaining powder time. He had come to Columbia after four weeks of steady decline that began with what he thought was a strep throat. He had become weak, short of breath, then was diagnosed with acute heart failure. His heart was dangerously enlarged, and an LVAD was our only hope of keeping Kory going until we could find a donor replacement.

I operated all day and spent an entire evening with the kid, struggling to keep him alive. Afterward, my legs ached, my arms and shoulders drooped, my eyeballs felt like lead weights. But more than the physical strain and fatigue, I was drained by the emotional stress, thinking that my young patient might die.

When I finally had a chance to slip away from Kory, who was now in his ICU room in somewhat stable condition, I dragged myself to my office. To get my mind and body ready to relax, I bent over at the waist, hanging my head down for a moment, then went into the yoga "down-dog" pose. My hips were in the air, my back was arched, my hands and feet were flat on the floor, my legs locked at the joints. I was in this position for maybe five minutes, just starting to ease down emotionally, when the phone rang. "Mehmet," said one of our most experienced anesthesiologists, Doug Jackson, "this kid's dying. He's not going to survive the way he is right now."

"Why?" I asked. "What's going on?"

"He's just progressively sinking."

Kory's main problem now was that the blood-flow rate, or outflow, of his new piggyback pump was very low. Not enough blood was being pushed out and across his lungs for oxygenation. My only option was to take Kory back to the OR to put in yet another pump. As I entered the ICU, I saw a crowd of about ten people in hospital smocks and scrubs gathered around Kory's bed—a bad sign. "What's up?" I said. They all snapped around to face me, hoping I could work some miracle and save the kid. Unfortunately, I was as uncertain as they were. I just tried not to show my despair.

Kory had a respirator tube inserted through his blue lips and taped to his bloated face, but the oxygen-saturation monitor was disturbing. The higher the pitch it emits, the healthier the patient's breathing and oxygenation. The lower the pitch, the sicker the patient. At that moment, Kory's vitals were playing the ominous four notes of Beethoven's Fifth. He looked as if he were about to die.

Suddenly, I remembered my father-in-law's notions about lymphatics and foot massage. If it works for dogs, I thought, maybe it'll work for humans. So I moved around to the foot of

Kory's bed, uncovered his feet, and without a word of explanation started to rub and squeeze them. Everybody stared—
the other doctors, nurses, the whole team—wondering what on
earth I was doing. But in a few minutes Kory's blood flows started
rising, from 2.1 liters per minute to 2.3, then to 2.5, up and up.
Whenever I quit squeezing, the flows would drop; when I started
again, they'd rise. So I kept it up for about forty-five minutes,
squeezing, rubbing, kneading the soles of his feet, milking the
lymphatics until his flows stayed up at a healthy level. Kory had
just needed to be jump-started toward recovery.

Now, there are three ways to explain what happened: First,
maybe Kory's blood flows were about to go up anyway. Second, maybe I was squeezing his feet so hard that I "woke up" his
body, and it started pushing blood around. Third, maybe my
treatment actually worked. Can I prove my amateur reflexology
caused his turnaround? No, not on the basis of one case. But unless the trials we do in the future on reflexology prove otherwise,
I believe what happened to Kory was not a coincidence.

Formally trained practitioners of reflexology generally follow
methods developed in the early twentieth century from the work
of two Americans, Dr. William Fitzgerald and Eunice Ingham.
Fitzgerald first proposed that the human body was divided into
ten equal zones, extending from the top of the head to the toes.
He believed that stimulating a specific zone, or site, of the foot
could produce a desirable effect in a corresponding zone in another part of the body. Eunice Ingham later developed a "body
chart," which she claimed showed how every part of the body
was reflected at target sites on the soles, toes, and sides of the
feet. For example, the underside base of the big toe is closely
connected to the neck, and the central part of the sole next to
the ball of the foot reflects the heart.

Recent studies have demonstrated that when the acupressure
point for the eyes is pressed, a dynamic magnetic resonance scan
will show changes in the eye center of the brain. Perhaps this
may be a mechanism of action for these ancient treatments.

A complete reflexology treatment often takes thirty minutes to an hour. Practitioners relax both feet at the same time by stroking them. Starting with the toes, they work down to the heel, gradually covering the soles, top, and sides. When applying pressure to specific reflex sites, they rub, rotate, and press with their hands. Immediately after a session patients usually report a feeling of lightness and relaxation, sometimes even mentioning a kind of "release" in the area needing treatment.

Whether a practitioner touches the feet or the rest of the body, massage is essentially a tactile treatment. However, another sense is often involved: smell. Throughout the ages people have used aromatic oils and herbs to enhance massage. In the modern era this allied healing practice called aromatherapy—though still controversial—is fast becoming an accepted part of the complementary medicine arsenal. Like most complementary therapies, aromatherapy affects the entire body, improving general health and well-being. But its practitioners report that it can also be effective for specific chronic ailments, such as muscular and rheumatic pains, acne and other skin conditions, digestive disorders, and problems connected to menopause and postnatal illness.

Our sense of smell, located in the catacombs of the most primitive part of the brain, is extremely powerful. When we smell, our autonomic nervous system—our body's autopilot—can produce all kinds of physical reactions. The amygdala, the brain's emotional center, is directly connected to the olfactory gland, probably the most poorly understood gland in the body. The seat of human rage is also found in the amygdala, and an angry temperament—as we know—contributes to heart disease.

For Jane Buckle, who trained for years at Cambridge University and is now a consultant and practitioner in our Complementary Care Center, aromatherapy is not just the application of scents. Of the dozens of essential oils derived from plants, each has its own characteristic aroma and therapeutic properties—and so each fragrance affects the olfactory gland with different combinations of chemicals. Applied on the skin or sampled in whiffs in or near the nasal passages, some fragrances soothe and relax, while others stimulate and invigorate. Research at Duke University, for example, has demonstrated that the use of vanilla scent, administered nasally by catheter, can reduce the sensation of pain. Spicy smells, by contrast, heighten the response to pain. Aromatherapists also use fragrances to alleviate various mental states: marjoram, for instance, eases anxiety; jasmine lifts depression; and peppermint stirs mental concentration.

Essential oils are made by pressing and distilling natural plant material in order to yield a highly concentrated essence of the plant's fragrance. On average, an essential oil is seventy times more fragrant than the non-distilled plant it is made from. Because they are so highly concentrated, essential oils are rarely used directly on the skin but are added in very small quantities—typically 2.5 to 3 parts to a hundred—to a vegetable base oil.

Jane Buckle, with her years of know-how and kits of tiny vials, helped us devise studies on student volunteers to see if aromatherapy could benefit patients. By using aromatic oils rubbed onto the feet, we have been able to alter the heart rate variability, which shows that scents can affect the body's autonomic nervous system. During the study, we also discovered that American youths unlike adults in Asia, for example, where massage is commonplace—tended to become nervous or apprehensive when being rubbed with oils rather than inhaling them through nasal tubes or on gauze pads. In our next controlled studies, we'll probably use nasal methods of administration as we try to answer the question, "Can aromatherapy reduce postoperative tension and speed recovery in patients?"

And maybe we'll discover a whole lexicon of effective treatments.

7

Making Waves

The purpose of healing
is to bring us in harmony
with ourselves.

—O. Carl Simonton

Early in my experience with complementary medicine, I received a call from a woman who introduced herself us an energy healer and a graduate student in the school of public health. Julie Motz had heard I was interested in offering my patients— especially those with LVADs—more than the usual mix of drugs, surgical skills, and physical therapy that modern hospitals use to fight illness and disease. "Could we talk sometime?" Julie asked, and I quickly answered, "Sure, let's meet."

The words "energy healer" set off no alarms. I knew *energy healing*, or energy-oriented therapies, was an umbrella term that included many kinds of treatments, from acupuncture and homeopathy to therapeutic touch and various kinds of massage. Most of these approaches spring from ancient medical traditions in China and India, and are based on the belief that humans are physical beings as well as systems of energy that determine a person's mental, emotional, and spiritual health, or balance.

Practitioners believe that energy flows within the body through channels called *meridians*, with seven main energy centers or *chakras* (a Sanskrit word for wheel), aligned along the spine. Each chakra emits and absorbs a different *life force* (the Chinese call this *qi,* or *chi*), and it governs different areas, even organs, in the body. Removing blockages of the life force along the meridians, creating balance and dispelling illness, is the goal of energy healers. Many of them even claim to see subtle electromagnetic waves, or glowing auras, emanating from people, and these too indicate blockage sites.

When Julie came by for our meeting, I was immediately taken by her quick intelligence and articulate speech. She bubbled with ideas and appeared to have depth in a lot of areas, not all medical. Slightly built, with short hair and a soft-featured face, she smiled a lot and spoke with confidence. And she always wore extravagant hats, eventually earning her the nickname "The Sombrero Woman" from my colleagues.

At the time I had no idea if I would ever actually use her or any of the other self-proclaimed energy healers in a hospital setting. The Julies of the world have no formal credentials, and even though I was running my own program with the LVADs, I was already attracting curious stares from my colleagues for even meeting with someone they probably considered in the New Age orbit. Fortunately, some of my fellow surgeons, like Craig Smith, were fair skeptics. Craig, who is as diligent a surgeon as he is a hard-nosed scientist, supported my forays into complementary medicine, while insisting that everything we used be rigorously tested. For him as well as me, hard data was the best convincer.

I had begun to submit research protocols for studies on hypnosis, music therapy, aromatherapy and therapeutic touch—with sage advice from Don Kornfeld, the head of Columbia University's review board—but my efforts were meeting with limited success. Then one day the solution struck me. I was seeing a female patient who wanted her hair done, much the way my wife, Lisa, wanted a massage in the maternity ward. Of course, I could bring in a hairdresser as an "amenity," so why couldn't I also classify complementary medicine practitioners as amenities, people

who could offer patients breaks from the boredom that blan-
keted their lives in the hospital? But as an amenity, Julie could
not be paid by the hospital.

"So," I told her, "you'll have to come in on a voluntary basis,
like a candy striper or a priest."

"Great," she said, "when do I start?"

My patients loved her. It wasn't long before one patient
wanted Julie to accompany him into the operating room. George
Serafin was convinced that her work had made a difference in
how he felt and in his growing confidence that he would survive
his medical ordeal. It is highly unconventional for anyone other
than the surgical team to be admitted to the OR during a transplant, but I decided to make an exception, because of George's
extraordinary history and intense conviction about Julie.

When I first saw George, he looked like a puffy corpse with
vital signs that nearly matched his appearance. Under the fluo-
rescent lights of his hospital room, the skin of the forty-six-year-
old executive appeared doughy and swollen. The only sign of life
was his open, steady eyes. Display screens beeped, a computer-
ized heart monitor rolled out EKG paper, nurses gave their reports, and outside in the hallway a cardiologist opined that
George might well be on his way to the morgue.

A survivor of open-heart surgery ten years before, George
was now afflicted with end-stage heart disease. He had delayed
coming to the hospital so long that even a potentially lifesaving
heart transplant could not be done. He was even beyond the
help of a mechanical pump. His kidneys had shut down, and his
body was so waterlogged that when I pressed my fingers into his
shin, I left five inch-deep depressions in his skin. George even
admitted that he felt a chill, the first warning of the infection
that would probably take his life.

As I prepared my thoughts before making the grim an-
nouncement to the family, I took the precaution of having his
wife sit down. Then I carefully told of the misery and sure death
that would result even if we went ahead and inserted an LVAD.

Then I visited George's room, found him awake, and gave him the dire prediction. He listened to me patiently, then told me he had faced death before in Vietnam. A navy veteran, he had survived security missions under fire and felt he could tell when his number was up. "I'll know when death's time has come," he said, "and this is not it."

Surgeons know that patients who are sure they will die during surgery are all too often correct. But I wasn't sure if the reverse was true.

"George," I said, "I think it's too far gone."

"Doc," George said, "I'm not going to die. I know I won't. I have too much to live for."

So I brought in the LVAD team—nurses, physician's assistants, cardiologists, and social workers—to help determine the most rational course. But with George Serafin our normal criteria seemed irrelevant. He was so determined, so certain he would not die, that I decided to go ahead with the operation the next morning.

Gowned, gloved, and masked, I stood beside George's prone and anesthetized body. Our head nurse slapped the scalpel handle into my hand, and I made the initial skin incision from the top of the breastbone down to the navel. The OR phone rang. Microbiology was calling. The blood culture drawn during George's chill the night before had already grown bacteria. Normally this ominous sign would have cancelled the surgery, but the operation was already under way.

I continued, opening a space above the peritoneum—the sac containing the intestines, stomach, and liver—to implant the LVAD pump. Next, I used a surgical jigsaw to cut through the sternum, exposing the chest cavity and eventually George's enormous, melon-size heart. I then diverted the blood from the heart into the heart-lung bypass machine. His lungs were now deflated, his heart halted, and for several hours he was kept alive by the heart-lung machine. I stitched the LVAD tubes into the corresponding heart openings, and turned on the device. Off the heart-lung machine, George's pump-aided heart started up again.

But his battle had only just begun. Scar tissue from a prior bypass operation and liver damage from his failing heart led to torrential bleeding—a problem I could not stop. I put bone wax on the sternum to reduce the ooze. I added concentrated clotting factors from other patients onto the wound. I transfused blood-clotting factors and platelets. I took package gauze and put manual pressure on every bleeding site I could find. George still bled. I left his chest open for three days, operating every day to stop the bleeding. George remained unconscious with a breathing tube in place. On the third day the bleeding finally stopped. George was still alive—not by much, but holding on.

The next morning George regained consciousness. As I examined him, I smiled, thinking of all the heroics performed on his body, but I didn't tell him of the war we'd waged. Later he asked me, and I described what happened. He smiled, then he shocked me. "That's what I thought," he said, adding that for three days he had felt as if he'd been swimming through a thick soup that buoyed him up but also made his movements difficult. His head also seemed heavy, yet he saw a bright light overhead. He thought that if he could just stay under the light he would live. Each time the light moved, he would maneuver himself back into the center. Finally, the light didn't move; he was safe.

"You remember that?" I asked him.

"That's *all* I remember," George said. "I kept thinking, 'I'm not dead yet. I have to get back under the light. I do that and I'll be all right.'"

While awaiting a donor heart, George began treatments with Julie. She had asked me to run through everything that my surgical team and I would do to George, so she could take him through the surgery step by step on an emotional level. I had seen how she had greatly lowered anxieties in other patients. We had given them questionnaires asking them to evaluate how energetic and anxious they felt before and after Julie's treatments.

Almost invariably they claimed to feel more energetic and less tense with the sessions.

So when I replaced George's old diseased heart and the pump, Julie was there, gowned and masked like the rest of us. She first positioned herself at his feet, and with her eyes closed, she rubbed and squeezed them, looking as if she were in some altered state herself. Later she moved to his head, keeping her hands floating a few inches over his forehead, never distracting me or interfering with surgical procedures. Actually, during the entire struggle to transplant George safely, I was so riveted on my trouble-shooting tactics that I hardly noticed Julie and her ministrations. Only when the surgery was long over, after she asked George to "welcome" his new heart with words of appreciation, did she tell me her unique interpretation of the operation.

"For him it was like running a marathon," she said.

"I know the feeling. I've run a few myself."

"His body was really struggling," she continued, "working just as hard as you. He never gave up. That's why he's so tired now. It's not because of the anesthesia." She added that she had seen George in the pre-op waiting room, and he seemed to have a confident grip on the ordeal ahead. In the OR, because George had renal insufficiency, she focused on his kidneys—using the energy emanating from her hands to shift and ease the energy "blockage" in his kidneys. Later, he boasted that his urine output had risen.

For Julie, and increasingly for me, getting to know a patient was less a matter of connecting the dots from what I read on a chart than it was "reading" a patient's emotions. A person's medical history, the vital stats, the opening of the chest, seeing the effects of nicotine or a fat-heavy diet—these were so many external facts. Her assessment of a patient's internal or emotional life, the distresses of grief, anger, loneliness, or ongoing pain—this she would pass on to me as an additional guide in healing.

George is now back to a normal life, running his own business. "Before all this happened," he told me, "I never went to church. Now I go every Sunday. I've got my life back."

I explained my initial reservations about operating and my very human limitations as a surgeon. "Sometimes," I added, "it's better to be lucky than good, although I like to be both."

George shook his head. "Naw, Doc," he said. "See, I just don't quit. I don't know the word."

Every clinician has cases that defy easy explanation. Usually, we mumble something about luck or chance, shake our head, and move on to the next patient. But George's story and Julie's role in it stuck in my mind. As she reminded me, I should never underestimate the effect of a patient's willpower on the body.

"I believe emotions are of the body, not of the brain," Julie would say. "Fear, anger, love, pain—they occur in the body. Too much repressed anger, and the result is depression and illness. Anger is the emotion that most affects the heart." In turn I mentioned studies that confirmed the depression–heart-disease link, including the observation that depressed patients have higher levels of stress hormones in the blood than those in non-depressed people. This results in higher blood pressure, a speeded up heart rate, and blood that clots more easily—all factors contributing to major cardiac problems. Moreover, depressed patients produce higher levels of cortisol, which can exacerbate the erratic heartbeats that often precede sudden death. Cortisol also decreases the secretion of growth hormone, which shifts the body's cholesterol toward the dangerous low-density lipoproteins (blood fats) and away from the high-density ones that protect blood vessels.

Then Julie explained that sometimes during sessions she would get visions or images of great sadness. She explained that healing occurs through relationships, which for her often means physically touching patients—a technique that other energy healers, like therapeutic touch practitioners, don't feel is necessary. "When I touch people," she explained, "I feel things. It's not hot or cold. It's more like a tingling and a pressure. I don't have to touch. I *like* to touch. Patients in hospitals are terribly touch-deprived."

Julie also insisted that I should talk to my patients during surgery. If I (and probably most surgeons) don't mutter words, even prayers and pleas, under our breath to our patients, we direct thoughts to them. I remember as a med school student watching my father-in-law in the OR. Gerald Lemole, a famous heart surgeon, would tell his unconscious patients to get their hearts to beat stronger and to stop bleeding. He would pretend to say this tongue in cheek, but I think deep down he was serious.

I was also meeting with scientists who studied energy healing and was impressed that a genuine effort was being made to determine whether or not these phenomena existed. Glen Rein, a Ph.D. at Quantum Biology Research Labs in Northport, New York, had made inroads into breaking what he believed to be energy phenomena into discernible categories in order to make them easier to investigate. Daniel Benor, a New Jersey physician, psychotherapist, and energy-healing researcher, was investigating therapeutic touch, a fast-growing healing field especially favored by nurses. Commonly known as "laying on of hands," therapeutic touch is based on the principle that the energy of our bodies extends beyond the boundaries of our skin. Though methods vary, a practitioner's goal is to unblock any congestion in the patient's energy field so that natural healing abilities of the body can function better. The therapist also balances and energizes the body through a series of rhythmical, sweeping hand movements a few inches from the skin, as if to "smooth out the wrinkles" in the patient's energy field.

Dr. Benor estimates that at least thirty thousand nurses and other caregivers practice therapeutic touch in the United States and more than eight thousand such healers are registered in the United Kingdom to give treatments in hospitals at the request of patients. British hospital centers for cardiac rehabilitation and for treatment of pain and cancer use these healers regularly. In

Eastern Europe and Russia, this kind of therapy increasingly is integrated with modern allopathic treatment. Although energy healing appears at odds with conventional scientific views, Dr. Benor believes that as rigorous, convincing research into energy medicine spreads, this ancient healing approach will gain wider acceptance by the mainstream medical community.

Can we really emit energy from our hands? We know that nerves transmit electrical pulses, and we know that electric currents give off electromagnetic fields. We also know that each thought comes about in a separate pattern of neurons firing. So why is it so hard to go the next step—at least to speculate that each thought produces a different state of energy? And why can't that energy be transferred out of the body? I feel encouraged in this sentiment by my exposure to energy healers from other cultures. One particularly revealing experience occurred after I gave a talk at the well-respected American hospital in Istanbul. My father and Eric Rose were with me, and just as we were getting ready to leave the lecture hall, I felt a tap on my elbow. "Dr. Oz, there's a woman outside who would like to meet you," a polite, male voice said in Turkish. "She's an energy healer. Would you have a few minutes?"

"Lead the way," I said.

Her name was Nurcan and she came from Azerbaijan, one of the Turkish-speaking Russian republics bordering northeast Turkey. About thirty-five, Nurcan said she had studied the same allopathic system of medicine that I and my colleagues had studied. So with ease she could speak the language of today's biology, organic chemistry, anatomy, and physiology. After her conventional medical training in Moscow, she said she studied energy healing for several years before moving to Turkey. I was intrigued. I had never met anyone who was trained in both the new and old medical worlds.

Eric volunteered for a treatment. Nurcan had him lie down on a sturdy, padded table, then paused to concentrate her thoughts. Throughout the session I translated her Turkish words, trying to imitate her soft, soothing tone. "Now, turn over . . . lie on your back. Close your eyes . . . let your arms and legs relax . . . feel your hands and feet go heavy. . . ." Eric remained quiet, expressionless. Nurcan began moving her outstretched arms an inch or two above his body, almost touching his skin. The small, delicate hands made discreet circular movements, sometimes pausing over certain spots.

As she later explained, a person's energy field extends beyond the skin, like an invisible aura. Nurcan apparently was directing *her* energy through her hands into the clogged-up, warmer areas where the energy was not flowing properly—that is, was not in balance or in harmony with the rest of the body.

Eric seemed to have fallen asleep by the time she finished. He opened his eyes. After a moment he sat up, smiled at my father and me, and said, "This isn't what I expected. It's far from anything in Western medicine." I asked him how he felt, and he answered, "Great! I don't know how it would affect other people, but whatever it is, it's relaxing."

Then Nurcan demonstrated the use of her "energy rod," a two-foot-long, straight piece of coat hanger-type wire with an inch or so at one end bent sharply away at a ninety-degree angle. She held the wire by the angled tip, grasping it between a thumb and a forefinger. Then she slowly moved the wire downward over Eric's chest and abdomen while he was standing. She held it a few inches away from his clothes. Suddenly the tip of the wire moved into his right, upper abdomen. "His liver is weak," Nurcan said. I translated, and Eric joked it was probably too much good Turkish wine. Then I asked if I could try moving the wire over Eric, thinking she may have twirled the wire around by some trick. But I could not grasp the tip hard enough with just my thumb and finger to purposely twist the long wire—and when I reached the spot over his liver area, to my surprise the wire abruptly moved in as it had before.

Apparently the energy rod worked like a water-seeking dousing stick, yet none of us could come up with a rational explanation—at least in our terms—for what we had witnessed. We left Nurcan and her unusual diagnostic tool, amazed at what we had witnessed.

Angus McDonald was another patient of mine who tried therapeutic touch, with even more dramatic results. A middle-aged LVAD patient who eventually received a transplant, Angus approached his sojourn at the hospital determined to heal as well as he could. More than twenty years before, he had undergone a quadruple bypass, and now even with the LVAD, he was near death because his lungs were barely functioning. Angus had ARDS, or Adult Respiratory Distress Syndrome, which was first formally described during the Vietnam War. Badly wounded young soldiers would die, not from their wounds, but from "pneumonia"—except it wasn't pneumonia. It was this inflammatory condition, an irritation that affects the lungs of very sick people. ARDS is usually lethal, and that's what worried me about Angus McDonald.

Angus, like most men in the West, had reservations about energy medicine. He didn't know what to expect. But to me it seemed worth a try, even as an experiment. Two energy practitioners worked on him together. They had him lie down in his hospital bed flat on his back, telling him he could keep his eyes open if he wished. After that they extended their arms and hands above his body, one woman at his feet, the other at his head. Suddenly, he felt an intense heat and, looking up, saw a hand extended six to eight inches over his body. "Then came a rapid temperature change," he later told me, "sort of like what you feel when you put your hand near a hot iron. It was a lot more than a person's body could give off."

Of course, it's impossible for a hand, no matter how hot, to project that kind of heat. As the hand passed over his body, he felt the heat move with it. He closed his eyes again and then felt a cold sensation radiating down from the hand and a second patch of coolness on his face. Again, hands should not be able to transmit coldness through mere conduction. It's very difficult for a cold hand to affect another person's skin without touching it.

During the procedure Angus asked the practitioners how the hot-cold sensations really worked. "That's when I realized it was some kind of other energy," he said. "It was something with which I was completely unfamiliar, because the next thing I knew, I was seeing this pale blue light, a really light blue, when the cold hand came down. It looked like the light was between her hand and my eyes. And then it expanded. It was like I got an infusion of blue all around. An incredible, wonderful feeling."

Angus explained that the soft blue light would increase and decrease as the two women started or stopped moving their hands over him. The healer told him that pale blue was the color of the aura she was projecting. "Quite honestly," he told me, recalling that session, "I'm not sure how it was happening. I was not a strong believer in this. But I was stunned to see what effect it had."

"How did you feel afterward?" I asked.

"Extremely refreshed," he said. "It made me feel a whole lot better."

Not everyone treated by energy practitioners can detect auras and temperature changes as Angus did. Now, did I as his surgeon see any beneficial effect to him as a result of the treatments? Well, Angus did do well with the LVAD. He eventually got a new heart and went home to resume a normal life. But there was nothing spectacularly unexpected or too out of the ordinary in his recovery. He did say he believed the treatments helped his body avoid tissue rejection from the transplant. "No real proof," he said, "but that's what I was thinking."

As for auras and energy fields around the human body—the kind sensed by Angus McDonald—researchers are attempting to prove that they exist by using high-tech laboratory equipment to measure very subtle electromagnetic activity emanating from study subjects. But proving we can change these fields to affect other living organisms is another matter. In the past, if sick people were "cured" by the laying on of hands, the tendency was to attribute the cause to the placebo effect. People who *expected* to get well probably would. Reputable studies prove such cures do occur in one out of three cases. But until recently investigators haven't looked much at the expectations and feelings of the physician or practitioner during energy treatments.

Bernard Grad, now a retired biology professor at McGill University in Montreal and a longtime researcher in the field of bioenergetics, believes that persons who claim to have the gift of some kind of energy healing with their hands often say their work is not done by themselves but by a "higher power" to whom they are connected. This greater power is not necessarily God or a spiritual entity. Sometimes it is described in terms of a life force, energy flow, life energy, or universal connectedness held together by some as yet undefinable electromagnetic forces. In different cultures and creeds it has gone by different names— God, the Great Father, *prana*, *chi*. So in this sense the healer, therapist, or shaman serves as a helpful, caring, cheerful, even loving conduit of such a greater power.

In well-documented experiments over more than three decades, Grad has tested the laying-on-of-hands effects with lab animals, plants, yeast, and inanimate objects. In one experiment, a practitioner's treatment significantly slowed the growth of goiters in mice. In another, carefully controlled experiment, repeated treatments speeded the healing of wounds in another set of mice. In this trial he made skin wounds on the backs of three sets of mice. A researcher twice a day held one group in his hands; a second group, which served as control, was held in the hands of an energy healer, and the third group of mice was treated only with heat and not by holding. After five days the energy healer showed that he could significantly accelerate the healing process. There were three to four times as many healed wounds on the mice in the healer's group than in the control group and an even higher percentage when compared to the group treated with only heat.

Although Grad sheds little light on what might cause such effects in acceptable scientific terms, he reminds us that the observed effects cannot be explained solely in terms of any known physical or chemical forces. Nor can we point to a placebo reaction, since mice presumably are not suggestible the way humans are.

Valerie Hunt, another well-known researcher in the bio-energy field, claims to have successfully measured the presence and the different, changing colors of human energy fields. Trained in neurophysiology with teaching credits at Columbia and UCLA, Hunt has used sensors and measuring devices that pick up extremely high-frequency waves of electricity—beyond the frequencies of muscle, brain, and heart electricities—and she has correlated these electromagnetic waves that surround the body with auras.

In Hunt's studies, healers would look independently at one set of patients, and all would separately describe a blue aura. With other patients the healers would all describe a yellow aura, or a light-colored mist, or maybe a dark-colored glow. These auras, or coronas, are invisible to most people and can extend five to ten feet away from the body. At all times, Hunt reported, this visible sign of the energy force within and around the body was constant and continuous.

People who claim to be able to see auras often say they can "scan" the body's energy field, sensing areas of heat, cold, pain, soreness, numbness, and tingling. A few say they can actually see and interpret the colors of auras, picking up the effects of past injuries and potential, future traumas. Some even believe they can do this at great distances by meditating on a name or touching a photograph of the target subject.

Even more mainstream scientists have been able to make radiographic images of people, revealing very small energy fields around them. Every one of our cells has energy. As a matter of fact, our bodies work only because our cells have energy gradients, or changing rates of ion flow across their surfaces. The reason some electrolytes stay in and some stay out is based on energy fields. It's critical to keep these energies separate. If, for example, sodium is not kept outside the cell and potassium kept inside, you would not have a live cell. That's the whole foundation of life—the ability of the cell membrane to keep the outside world separate from the inner cell.

In our clinic we attempted to test if energy healers could actually control the energy they emitted. To do so, we used a high-voltage electrophotographic process known as Kirlian photography, named for an eccentric Russian scientist who in the 1930s found that "coronas" or haloes of light were visible around people's fingers that were placed near high-voltage electric fields. Most of the extensive Soviet literature in this field, deemed confidential by the Russian government, has never been released in the West; and so we had to develop our own Kirlian "camera."

The principle of Kirlian photography is simple. All matter, including human beings, have electrons spinning around atoms, which are the building blocks of all things. If our hands get close to a strong electric field, some of the electrons in the surface of our skin will be pulled away and will jump ship, so to speak, to head for the more magnetic force of the electric field. During their travels the electrons will collide with anything in their path, including electrons of other atoms. When they do hit another electron, they give it more energy, which is called "exciting it" to a higher state. When the "excited" electrons eventually relax, they throw off their extra energy in the form of photons, which have characteristic visible hues that can be photographed. Since most of the collisions the electrons make will be with nitrogen, the most common gas found in air, Kirlian images usually appear blue-violet, which is the color nitrogen emits.

If energy healers could control the energy they emitted, we reasoned that any energy shifts they effected should be visible in their coronas. To create the technology we needed, we recruited Mark Russo, a confident, tough-nosed engineer who learned his trade developing stealth weapons, to build the high-voltage electromagnetic plate, and Asim Choudhri, a top-notch biochemist-computer hacker in my lab, to analyze the color compositions of the coronas. We then pitted a group of energy healers against an equal number of untrained "control" subjects.

Mark found that every individual we tested emitted a characteristic halo of colors as his or her middle finger touched the electromagnetic plate. Asim scanned each halo into the computer, which broke its color down into the three primary component hues (red, yellow, and blue), and then further divided each hue into 256 categories of "deepness" to give us an exact "energy fingerprint" of each subject. We then asked our subjects to try consciously to alter their coronas. None of the untrained control subjects could do so, but in the energy healer group there were some subjects who were indeed able to change the color of their haloes, usually by intensifying the middle ranges of the color blue.

We repeated the study dozens of times to ensure that the subjects, not some fluke, were really changing the colors of their haloes and proved that the chance of these changes being pure coincidence was less than one in a thousand. We even tried to identify a physiologic cause of the changes by examining the effects of temperature, blood pressure, and intensity of finger pressure on the images. Even breathing fast, holding one's breath, or using biofeedback techniques could not cause changes.

So we know that some trained energy workers can alter the energy in ways we do not understand. This does not mean that the alterations lead to any healing, but at least we now have a jumping-off point on which to base further studies.

Much of the pioneering research into electromagnetic energy in the non-biological as well as biological worlds was done in the 1980s by Dr. Bjorn Nordenstrom, who was chairman of radiology at the Karolinska Institute and Hospital in Stockholm. Nordenstrom's experiments have attempted to demonstrate the existence of a structured flow of electricity in the form of what he calls "biologically closed electric circuits," or fields, in living organisms. These systems of three-dimensional spirals or vortices vary in size and are dominated by a flow of positive and negative ions in circulating fields—much the same as electrical current is conducted through metal in varying wavelengths and amplitudes. Energy practitioners, of course, usually refer to chakras, the main energy centers in the human body, as "vortices."

More recently other scientists have injected radioactive isotopes into a person's "snuffbox"—the flesh part of the hand between thumb and index finger—and have been able to track through X-ray pictures the isotopes' movement along energy *meridians*, not along any pathway system identified in Western medicine. That is, an acupuncturist trained in the traditional Chinese way of mapping body energy could predict how isotopes would flow from the hand toward the body core more accurately than a Western-trained doctor.

A well-documented, controlled study done in Shanghai shows how the use of these energy meridians by acupuncturists can help cardiac-surgery patients. Anesthetized by needles expertly placed at specific meridian points in the ears and extremities, 107 patients were found after surgery to have a "marked reduction or the absence of various post-operative respiratory symptoms and complications." Scandanavian researcher Soren Ballegaard has published impressive results when acupuncture is used to relieve angina in patients who are not candidates for more traditional remedies. In the United States, acupuncture and the use of energy meridians to promote pain relief and healing has found widespread acceptance. But as of now acupuncture is still the only energy-based technique approved for use in American hospitals, though mostly to treat substance-abuse patients.

One big question my lab researchers and I are trying to answer is how energy healing might affect cellular activity, particularly in immune and cancer cells. Such research might sound far-fetched, or even preposterous, but our first "small-question" efforts are very encouraging. Of course, within the conventional medical establishment the mere existence of such a phenomenon as energy healing is usually greeted with disbelief. Mostly this is because all attempts to measure the actual energy transfer—at least as published in Western medical literature—have failed. Part of the reason may be that any measurement system to assay energy medicine inevitably affects the energy. In physics this is called the Heisenberg uncertainty principle. Physicists recognized in the 1920s that if you described the nature of electrons by bouncing other electrons off them, the path of the investigated particle would necessarily be changed by the investigation. Consequently, the direct measurement techniques we use to gauge the subtle powers of energy medicine may overwhelm the energy-healing treatments we use. For this reason we elected to use a biologic-model assay—an indirect means of assessing the vitality of energy medicine.

Under strict scientific controls, Frank Huo, an energy healer trained in China, and three other practitioners, two of whom use therapeutic-touch techniques, treated breast-cancer cells grown in petri dishes. Frank repeatedly demonstrated he could affect, or slow, cancerous growth, albeit to a very small degree, while the other practitioners produced interesting yet less consistent results. Frank appeared to be doing something exceptional to these normally explosive, super-aggressive cells.

Sonal Shah, a promising researcher in my lab, took charge of running the experiments with Frank and the others. A top graduate of Brown University with a degree in philosophy, she will soon follow her parents into some field of medicine (her father's a surgeon, her mother a molecular biologist). "I'm very much a skeptic about energy healing," Sonal said straightaway when I first asked her to help out. I told her I preferred a hard science-oriented, rigorous approach to the work.

In one of the equipment-crowded lab rooms of the hospital's research building, Sonal grew the cancer cells in an incubator in small, covered glass containers filled with a pink-colored nutrient that looked like Kool-Aid. Normal cells are social and chummy with their neighbors. When they get to a certain density, they stop growing. However, tumor cells simply grow and grow and grow. They're like weeds, very asocial, pushing out all other growth, crowding, fighting for space.

Sonal would take samples of these cells and, using a grid of tiny squares, count them under a microscope before and after the energy treatments. Separately, she would show Frank and the others into a quiet testing room where they would perform their treatment, while standing. Frank, eyes closed, his hands one over the other and about six to ten inches above the glass container with the cells, was particularly intense during the half-hour to one hour sessions. Each practitioner used a particular word or phrase as they focused on emitting energy, or *chi*, through their hands. Frank's method was to concentrate on clearing his mind of all thought except the word *kill*.

A young, bright-eyed native of Beijing, Frank Huo has studied the mind-body-energy techniques of "Yuanji science" for many years. Incorporating elements of Taoism, Buddhism, and Confucianism, this way of life for achieving harmony, kindness, and good health also involves harnessing the body's natural energy system. What Frank was doing with the cells, he says, was simply using his energy to bring about harmony—in this case, to kill a destructive uncontrolled part of life. He was operating much like China's *chi-gong* masters, who reportedly can move or affect inanimate objects without touching them. Dr. David Eisenberg, an instructor in medicine at the Harvard Medical School, has described one such demonstration of energy force. While in China he watched a *chi-gong* master breathe deeply three or four times, then point one foot and a hand at a heavy, cut-glass, hanging lantern, which suddenly began to sway back and forth. The *chi-gong* master was three feet away from the lantern, and Eisenberg was convinced he was not tricked.

In our second test, Sonal looked at how frequently thymidine, a radio-labeled nucleotide, is incorporated into the cancer cells. The faster the cells grew, the more thymidine was absorbed.

When we compared the "energy treated" cells with control-group cells that had no energy treatment, we also found somewhat faster growth in the untreated cells. We're now doing more sophisticated tests, by treating human, disease-fighting lymphocytes with energy in order to find out whether they kill a given antigen more or less frequently. If we discover energy does fight cancer—at least outside the body in a petri dish—then we'll see how Frank's treatments affect cancer patients *inside* their body. This will be our final series of "small" questions we'll ask to answer the big query, "Can energy healing cure cancer?"

The late science-historian Thomas Kuhn, in elaborating on his notion of paradigm shifts, argued that science doesn't evolve by making smooth, gradual progress with small, incremental steps. Rather, a new discovery or convincing research data forces scientists to view reality in a very different light. The field of mind-body energy may provide the catalyst for bringing on just such a shift in our vision of illness and the healing arts.

❧ 8 ❧

Spiritual Will

*Life is like a candle. The soul is the
flame licking towards the heavens;
the wick is the body holding us down.*

—Rebbe Menachem Schneerson,
as adapted by Simon Jacobson
and compiled by Steven Dubner

Most doctors—whether or not they admit it publicly—have encountered a hopeless, dying patient who somehow, inexplicably, survives. Inexplicable, unless you consider a strong dose of prayer—from loved ones, from strangers, from people nearby and faraway, requested or unsolicited. It's probably the oldest healing therapy in human history. Yet, as Dr. Larry Dossey, eloquent author and former chief of staff of Medical City Dallas Hospital, notes, it's "one of the best-kept secrets in modern medicine."

Surveys show that of all the unconventional healing practices used in America, prayer is by far the most common—employed by 91 percent of women, 85 percent of men. Among the patients admitted to our heart service, most consider prayer to be their only method of complementary medicine.

And, as Dossey and others have argued, prayer can work. Dr. Randolph Byrd, a cardiologist at the University of California Medical School at San Francisco, studied nearly four hundred patients suspected of having heart attacks. They were divided roughly into two, randomized groups, both being given state-of-the-art medical treatment. The first names of those in one group were given to various Protestant and Catholic groups who were asked to pray for these patients. Neither the doctors and nurses nor the patients knew who was or was not being prayed for.

The patients who were prayed for proved far less likely to develop congestive heart failure, five times less likely to require antibiotics, and three times less likely to need diuretics. Fewer of the prayed-for group caught pneumonia. It was as if the prayed-for group had been given a miracle drug!

And prayers from across the country seemed as effective as those from groups close to the hospital. Other controlled, published studies have compared the ability of people to influence the growth rates of organisms solely with their mind, both at close range (about an arm's length) and at distances up to fifteen miles. In these studies too, distance had been shown to be irrelevant; whether near or far, the strength of the influence was the same. Dossey and others have observed that such experiments in prayer-based healing give a consistent picture: prayer is not a conventional form of energy, like electricity, that diminishes in strength with distance. Nor is it a form of energy that is "sent" or "received." Although scientists still cannot explain how prayer works at a distance, future controlled, repeatable experiments in fields as dissimilar as quantum physics and clairvoyance may someday shed light on how such healing functions.

In Kory Boglarski's case I didn't need Dossey to remind me that of all the unconventional treatments available, perhaps prayer—and not only the foot massage I gave him—affected the boy's course of healing during his LVAD and heart-transplant experience. Coming from a strongly Catholic family, Kory said his parents and sister prayed for him constantly. His sister even took a semester off from college so she could be with him. "We've always been good Catholics," Peg, his stepmother, explained toward the end of Kory's hospital stay, "but all this has brought us closer to each other and to God." Every night Kory was in the hospital, before his parents would leave, they would all sit down together and recite the evening's prayers.

Of course, this didn't exempt Kory from periodic funks. I remember one time during his eight-month stay with us when he sank into a deep depression and begged his parents to just let him go home and die. Jack and Peg told their son that they needed him and that his job was to stay alive. "God has a purpose for you," Peg said. "You just have to stick around to fulfill it." Kory later told me that when he heard those words, it was as if "God had spoken to him directly," as if God had said that to his whole body. From then on he never had second thoughts. He knew what he had to do.

The night Kory got his heart, his mother was at a healing mass. When the family got the call from the transplant coordinator, they had to leave immediately, since it would take two and a half hours to get to the hospital. Kory and his father were just pulling out of the driveway when Peg drove up. "You must have been praying a lot," Kory told her. "I just got a heart!"

We shouldn't eliminate using whatever works, no matter how strange, ancient, or unexplainable—in Western terms—the treatment is. Science has only just begun to explain the mind-body connection. I'm convinced our generally smug world of modern allopathic medicine—girded by occasional tolerance for other healing approaches—must offer patients a whole menu of complementary therapies, some of which we are now testing with an eye to having them sanctioned for optional, general use in the hospital. In this sense, if some patients pray, the practice hardly needs approval. It's simply a bonus in their overall treatment, a reflection of their attitude toward their illness—and attitude is often a deciding factor in successful recovery.

At Columbia Presbyterian, pastoral services—prayers, counseling, and rituals—have been expanding in recent years, and many of us doctors are inviting the clergy in because few of us—only 35 percent—are comfortable offering patients spiritual support. But if we were only to call the clergy to perform last rites for the dying or critically ill—when everyone has given up—I believe that we would deprive patients of an opportunity to invoke yet another potential aid to their own healing.

I recall a particular patient I met from Texas, Gerald White. This sixty-six-year-old man had had a cancerous kidney removed and unfortunately developed a recurrence requiring a second operation a year later. Within four months of the renewed attempt to cure the cancer surgically, new growths appeared in his lungs, which were consistent with the spread of cancer. Mr. White was placed on an aggressive immunotherapy program, but this therapy, too, was ineffective in stemming the new growths.

After eight months of being "knocked down" by this treatment without success, Mr. White began to attend a prayer and healing session every Wednesday evening at an Episcopal church nearby. After combing the literature for self-help clues, he added meditation and guided imagery to his prayer regimen. Within four months the masses in the lungs had disappeared, and he has remained free of disease for nearly two years. His doctors cannot explain his recovery, which he attributes to prayer.

Sometimes faith alone can do the healing. Frank Jones, another LVAD patient, was a husky forty-five-year-old "sandman" who hauled and spread sand on roads and highways in upstate New York. During an especially heavy snowstorm he collapsed from exertion and had a massive heart attack that left him unconscious and near death. Several colleagues advised me that he was too far gone to save, but I had already met Frank's wife and children—an experience that generally compels me to operate even in the face of great odds.

The challenging operation was remarkably uneventful, and when Frank regained consciousness, I expected the usual outpouring of admiration for my team's work in the OR. But Frank was not only depressed because his heart had let him down, but upset at me for saving his life. "Dr. Oz," he said, "I was supposed to die. I was going to a better life. What use am I going to be to anybody now?"

I was taken aback by this reaction but thought he might soon change his mind. I was wrong. Over the next few weeks Frank stopped eating, lost weight, and in a sense became passively suicidal. I learned from a social worker that he was quite religious. So I brought in the big guns, his minister and his wife. We brainstormed and came up with a perfect game plan, one that could restore Frank's sense of purpose in life and one that he could not refuse. We managed to convince him that he was needed as an evangelist for his church. And now Frank rallied, saying that it was his duty to God to get well and do good work. Finding a meaningful purpose in life had renewed him.

For many patients, being treated in a hospital and having surgery is a big jump into the unknown. Paul Broadhead, for example, came to me for a heart transplant with a crusty, fix-me-up attitude. He was a self-made real estate tycoon who was used to being the boss. Though his heart was failing, he was still in his middle-age prime with big plans for the future. He seemed to treat his heart disease as just another bump in the road or a temporary delay before zipping back to work.

By the time his number came up and a donor was found, he was quite ill and at his most vulnerable. The words alternative, complementary, holistic, mind-body, spiritual—these were not in his vocabulary. "When something in the body is broken, you fix it, period," he would say. "You don't question the whys and hows of the disease. That's a chore for the guys in white lab coats."

So I had to convince him: "Believe me," I said, "patients do better if they play an active role. You should recover faster, and you can use these tools to continue your healing at home."

As I described our complementary therapies, the silver-haired mogul groused but then said he'd try some massage, yoga, and meditation exercises. But Paul Broadhead also had an amazing spiritual side. He told me he had made a two-decade study of near-death phenomena—and for a deeply personal reason. He said that eighteen years prior to my surgery on him, he had died on another OR table. He remembered slipping away euphorically to a brightly lit corner of the operation suite and watching his surgeon try to resuscitate him. He felt so "wonderful" he didn't want to return.

But then he had qualms about the well-being of his family, since he had left so many issues in his life unresolved. As his desire to live returned, he temporarily lost his vision, and for many years he felt awkward discussing this entire experience. As he approached my operation, he admitted that he had made plans for death. If the same bright-light situation occurred, he would choose to leave this world peacefully.

I had a similar experience myself, as a child. I was in my grandfather's wondrous garden in Turkey, peering into the depths of its magnificent goldfish pool. From above, magnified by the water, the fat, lazy-looking fish seemed the size of melons. Most were speckled orange, yellow, and black, but I saw one red fish, and I wanted him. I wanted to feel his plump flesh in my hand, touch his wavy little wings, look into his flat eyes. I wanted to know him, to understand what "fish" was.

So, carefully I reached into the water, where the red fish floated just below my grasp. Balancing my weight on the pool's edge, I stuck my entire arm in and almost touched him. Suddenly he darted away, and as I lurched after him, I tumbled head first into the deep water.

I was five years old and had no idea how to swim. Yet once the water closed over me, I was not afraid. Oddly I felt neither wet nor cold. It was as if I'd been engulfed by a liquid cloud that was so beautiful, soft, and utterly alien. Looking up, I could see the shimmering light at the surface and was mesmerized by the rippling patterns. I couldn't breathe, and for a moment I panicked, thrashing about as I sank to the bottom. But still I was transfixed by the beauty of my underwater haven, the colors, the play of light; and so I abandoned myself to the experience, feeling it and accepting it.

All at once the water seemed to darken. I felt a powerful hand clamp my wrist and yank me up and out of the pool. It was my mother who, ever watchful, had known better than to turn her back on her mischievous little boy. She saved me, but not before I had a glimpse of a kind of peace that could come with the end of life.

As a heart surgeon, I've encountered a number of patients who report such out-of-body experiences. One of them was Samye Isenberg, a practicing nurse married to a physician. I met her the day before her surgery. She was propped up on her pillows, her hands folded over her stomach. I introduced myself, outlined the procedure I would do the next morning, and went over the risks involved. It was a more complex case than the usual bypass operation and carried a higher chance of failure—a euphemism for death. But Samye did not appear to be concerned. I thought perhaps she didn't realize how serious her condition was.

"Oh, I know I might die," she replied in a chatty, upbeat tone. "I'm not worried about it."

I didn't know what to say. Most of my patients, whatever their religious beliefs, are at least a little anxious at the prospect of dying.

"You know," Samye said, "I've died twice already."

"What do you mean?" I asked, sitting at the foot of her bed.

"When I was four years old," she began, "I slipped under the water near our house by the Connecticut shore and started to drown. I remember voices around me, and I was raging to whatever force was pulling me away about how I was still a little girl and hadn't had a chance to live my life. I demanded another chance. I didn't know if anyone was listening, but my mother tells me I was pulled to the surface and was barely kept alive."

Another time, years later, she had a close call while receiving dye for a study of her kidneys. She had an anaphylactic reaction, the worst allergic reaction to have, and lost her blood pressure. This time Samye felt herself losing consciousness and then saw a blinding light. The next thing she knew, she was looking down at the resident who had given her the dye injection and other white-coated doctors frantically trying to bring her back. Eventually, they succeeded and Samye's out-of-body view faded and was lost.

Fascinated, I asked Samye if she had any other out-of-the-ordinary sensations.

"Yes," she said.

When she was seven she woke up in the middle of the night and told her mother that her Uncle Sidney had died. She could only explain that she "just knew." The next morning, her aunt called the family to tell them that her husband, Sidney, had dropped dead of a heart attack.

I've had other patients with LVADs who also exhibited what seems like telepathy. One, Betty Diotaiuti, was an unofficial "leader" of one of our groups. An upbeat, very determined, heavy-set woman in her early fifties, she had been waiting for a heart much longer than the others—for nearly a year—yet her spirits seldom dropped. For twenty years her enlarged-heart condition was kept in check with drugs; then one Christmas Eve her breathing became labored and she was so tired she could not walk. She had invited twenty-six people over for dinner and felt bad that she had to head for the hospital instead of baking the lasagna. A week and a half later, she was in cardiogenic failure and I implanted her pump.

But Betty couldn't stay idle. As soon as she was able, she began making styrofoam and plastic Christmas decorations and selling them at a small folding table in the hospital lobby. Then, not long before New Year's Eve, Betty started telling her friends and the nurses on duty that she was getting a heart transplant very soon. As Carol Ann, a superb veteran nurse, told me, "I was talking to Betty, and I mentioned that we might have champagne for a little New Year's Eve toast, and she said, 'I won't need it.' I asked her, 'Why not, don't you like champagne?' And she said, 'Oh, it's not that. It's because I'm going to be having a transplant.' I asked her how she knew, and she said it was just a feeling she had."

And sure enough, that night, after waiting almost a year Betty got her new heart.

We were all stunned. Consider what it takes to get a new heart: First, somebody within a sixty-mile radius of the hospital has to die, making a heart available roughly an hour after death. Then relatives of the deceased have to be willing to donate the organ, we among all the other transplanting hospitals have to qualify for the heart, and there can be no other patients in the region who are deemed more of a priority than Betty. Then we have to screen the donor, which had posed a problem for Betty because she had so many antibodies in her blood. Then, to make sure the heart will be compatible, we combine some of the donor's blood with Betty's. If Betty's antibodies don't kill the donor cells, then there is a chance she would not immediately kill the new heart after transplantation.

So many things had to happen for any transplant to happen. How could Betty have picked the day? I wasn't ready to accept her premonition as mere coincidence, but I couldn't explain it to myself in any scientific, logical way. I knew Betty as an open-eyed, feet-on-the-ground pragmatist, who had never made such "psychic" predictions before. Why pick a particular day—and no other day—with us to play clairvoyant?

Several months after Betty had her premonition, Maggie Palminteri had a similar experience. She spotted a small piece in *USA Today* indicating that if readers said a novena to St. Jude, patron of the impossible, their prayers would be answered. "You say the prayer nine times a day for a week," said Maggie, a Catholic but not a regular churchgoer. "So I prayed for a new heart. I just *believed*. I believed it would happen."

After a week of fervent praying, Maggie got her new heart. Was this just another coincidence? Or did Betty and Maggie have some higher state of consciousness that let them anticipate or affect major life events?

I don't generally think in such terms. I am a scientist, reliant on facts and statistics. But one of the first lessons surgery taught me was that medical science can be fallible.

Mr. Aja was a bear of a case: He'd had four previous open-heart surgeries, two mechanical hearts, and had hovered for months on the brink of death while awaiting a transplant. Finally, we got a donor heart for him. The surgery started out with major difficulties and got worse. Flora, our chief operating room nurse, should have handed me a chisel instead of a scalpel. I felt like a sculptor chipping out a heart from a chunk of granite. When we were done, the bleeding was torrential. For twenty hours straight we operated and were able to keep him alive only by artificially pumping liters of blood we were getting back into large-bore plastic catheters that we had inserted in his neck and arms.

The case had started in the pre-dawn hours, and finally at eleven that evening I told the exhausted, frustrated team that there was nothing more to be done. Mr. Aja was going to die. I closed him up, arranged for him to be moved from the OR, and went to speak to his wife. I explained that while we had been able to get him off bypass, we could do nothing to stop the bleeding. I expected he would pass away within several hours, certainly by morning. Leaving the team to make his last hours comfortable, I went home to await the end, and I advised the family to do the same after saying good-bye to him in his ICU room.

On those evenings when I lose a patient and leave the hospital through the big glass doors of the main entrance, the wind never seems as friendly as when I emerge triumphant from battle. That night a hot, humid gust moistened my face, and I started to sweat while walking through the August heat to the garage. I didn't sleep well that night, imagining myself snorkeling in the swells of blood that I hadn't been able to control in Mr. Aja's chest.

The next morning I was awakened by a phone call from a

highly agitated Mrs. Aja. Apparently, she had arranged for a mortician to come and pick up her husband, but the hospital refused to release his body. She asked that I take care of the matter. I immediately called the nurse in charge to see what the problem was.

"Bonnie," I said, "it's Dr. Oz. I'm calling about Mr. Aja."

"Hold on a second," Bonnie said. "I need to pull up his chart."

"No," I interrupted, "don't bother. I just want to find out why he hasn't been released."

"Excuse me?" She sounded genuinely puzzled.

"Why hasn't he been turned over to the morgue?" I asked. "His wife is really quite upset about the whole thing."

"Are you talking about your case from last night?"

I couldn't understand what was so difficult about my question. "Yes," I said. "Mr. Aja. His wife wants to get him over to the funeral parlor this morning."

Bonnie was quiet for a while, then giggled. I didn't see the humor in the situation. "But, Dr. Oz," she said, "Mr. Aja's not dead. He actually looks pretty good."

I was staggered by the news. Thrilled, but absolutely thrown, stunned. Every scientific indicator spelled certain death for Mr. Aja, but he had stopped bleeding after I left the ICU and had been improving through the night. To me, it was like revisiting the case of my Jehovah's Witness patient who survived against all possible odds. Call it fate, luck, karma, or providence—something beyond science had enabled these patients to live.

I began to study other healing systems. What I found remarkable in each, from Chinese acupuncture to homeopathy, from shamanism to therapeutic touch, was the concept that there exists a reality outside the physical realm—that life is dependent upon some force that is not discernible by any sensory method we acknowledge. This was what religion—which for the most part, I had resisted in any of its organized forms—had been saying all along.

I remember one of my surgical and spiritual mentors, Dr. Bashir Zikria, speaking of a surgeon's familiarity with death. A deeply religious Muslim, Dr. Zikria maintained that heart surgeons, because they literally take their patients' hearts in their hands, face death on very intimate terms and so have an actual tactile sense of the dividing line between matter and spirit. The heart is, after all, man's center point, the controller of his rhythm and pulse. In the surgeon's gloved palm lies the closest physical thing to the ethereal soul.

Most allopathic physicians don't take such a mystical view. Ironically, among all scientists it is physicists who have become most comfortable with addressing the aspects of the world that we cannot see, touch, or measure. As Fritjof Capra makes clear in his pioneering book *The Tao of Physics*, our perception of this other reality may be skewed by our personal limitations. For example, if I showed you a picture of two equal circles placed side by side and asked you what they represented, your first response probably would not be "a doughnut." However, if I explained that this was a doughnut cut across its diameter, not its circumference, and that the two cut ends of the resulting magnet-shaped half doughnut had been touched to the paper and traced, you would then be able to imagine a third dimension of the doughnut, depth. But what if I asked you to imagine the doughnut in *four* dimensions—that is, the fourth dimension being time? You would probably be stumped. Yet this way of viewing an object as something that exists in space *and* time is common in modern physics.

Eastern mystics, as Capra points out, seem to be able to attain non-ordinary states of consciousness in which they transcend the three-dimensional world of everyday life to experience a higher, multidimensional reality. Larry Dossey and others elegantly describe the "non-local" mind—that is, a mind that transcends the individual—as being an overriding spiritual oneness that binds us all. If each of us were a raindrop, we would have an identity that was unique but also effervescent, since we would eventually fall into and merge with the sea, which represents communal consciousness. Perhaps it is in this other realm where that "oneness" of many minds that Larry Dossey describes functions to connect us all.

The need to transcend the ego, to subjugate the individual will, is a central tenet of most of the major religions. As the Buddha said, "Though he should conquer a thousand men in the battlefield a thousand times, yet he, indeed, who would conquer himself is the noblest victor."

In Islam, as in Orthodox Judaism, this is achieved with strict discipline. The human will is made subordinate to the will of God through a specific code of behavior. In India yoga is used to "yoke" the mind, controlling it by focusing it on the external. Buddhists seeking Nirvana follow the "eightfold noble path," a combination of right thought and right action, to cast off desire. Whatever method the religion dictates, the spiritual goal is the same, true freedom and ultimate happiness—or in many religions, regeneration and rebirth on a higher plane.

Searching through many seemingly conflicting doctrines, I have found that the great teachers urge us to let go of our attachments chiefly in two realms of life—the same areas that I see wreaking havoc on my patients. The first is our love of the world, our passion for physical things, our unsatisfied desires that often lead to suffering. The second is the selfishness that justifies our negative thoughts and emotions toward others. Anger, contempt, hatred—these keep us chained to our lower selves. True freedom lies in overcoming these base loves and choosing to follow a higher path.

For my patients, true healing often emerges out of life changes that involve setting aside petty and destructive emotions and the acquisitive, mundane preoccupations of our physical world, in order to embrace a higher good. Watching their transformation, I often think of Colin Wilson's remark in *The Reality of the Visionary World*:

If we believe in nothing but the material world, we become victims of the narrowness of our own consciousness. We are victims trapped in triviality. Religion gave us a reason for trying to reach the stars—for creating the magnificent spires and arches of the Gothic cathedrals, the great masses of the Rennaisance composers, the stained glass of Chartres, the masterpieces of Michelangelo. Where there is a distance between heaven and earth, there is also a great vault in which the spirit can soar. When heaven descends to earth, poetry has to crawl on its hands and knees.

❧ 9 ❧

Choices

To avoid illness, eat less.
To have a long life, worry less.

—Chinese proverb

I once attended an American Heart Association meeting where among the dozens of addresses being presented was one by Dr. Dean Ornish, the well-known apostle of lifestyle changes as a way to slow and even reverse heart disease. The standing-room-only crowd of cardiologists, surgeons, and other attendees spilled out into the hallway, though the room was as large as a fair-sized college lecture hall. I squirmed my way forward, but caught only a glimpse of the slender, moustached figure presenting his views and data.

Ornish has since become a medical celebrity among the general public. His "Opening Your Heart Program" has been followed by many heart disease victims to "fix" their coronary problems. The remedy, Ornish says, is a process intended to last a lifetime. It calls for a demanding diet consisting of only ten percent fat, plus at least a half hour a day of aerobic exercise, an hour a day of such de-stressing exercises as yoga stretches, deep breathing, meditation, relaxation, and visualization, and regular group-support meetings. It's not an easy prescription, and it's not for everyone. But it's had impressive results in actually *reversing* coronary-artery blockages without surgery or drugs.

Back then, though, many physicians dismissed the importance of his data, saying that the amount of plaque reduction in the patients he studied was minuscule. Most of us knew his theories. We had seen his charts, graphs, numbers, and patient testimonies. A study he published showed that in twenty-eight people who adhered to a one-year program involving the lifestyle changes he prescribed, the average reversal was less than six percent at the end of a year. After four to five years of compliance, further reversal occurred—though the total still averaged only about eight percent.

However, these patients reported a *91 percent* reduction of angina (chest pains), a 55 percent improvement in their capacity to exercise, a 21 percent drop in cholesterol levels, and a marked decrease in blood pressure—even during emotional stress. They felt better and healthier, and PET scans, which show the blood supply to the heart muscles, showed evidence of improvement. But just as interesting to me was that while Dr. Ornish preached ancient methods, like diet and yoga, at the same time he seemed to represent a new and still developing way of looking at heart disease—a way that put the patient, not technology, in the driver's seat. Patients themselves had to choose to change—in what they ate, for instance—to reduce their risk of heart attacks. For Dean Ornish, how the heart functions as a result of certain lifestyle changes was just as important as the changes in the heart's structure. He viewed heart surgery mostly as a stopgap measure, with lifestyle changes being the real way to a long-term cure.

Ornish's promotion of yoga also caught my attention. I'd first been exposed to it one hot summer afternoon, when the Lemoles were visited by an old friend, Dr. Sandra McLanahan, who had worked with Dr. Dean Ornish in developing his pioneering program for coronary artery-disease reversal. Sandy gave me a mini-seminar on training the mind to focus while placing the body in age-old poses and stretches. As I lay facedown on the ground, arching my back in order to raise my face to the sky, I could fixate on continued, slow, repetitive breathing. No matter how uncomfortable the position, I stayed calm by focusing on my rhythmic, ever constant breathing. That afternoon, on the grass with the sun on my face, I did just about the entire routine of poses, and for me yoga worked. It was relaxing yet at the same time invigorating.

Yoga, which literally means *yoking* or *union*, is among the oldest known systems of health practiced today, originating in India probably about five thousand years ago. When I was in Bangkok, I saw animal figures that represented different yoga postures in Wat Po, a healing temple. Each pose represented a position that has therapeutic effects for organs or ailments. Houston Smith, the religious scholar, also has argued that these exercises depicted in stone, much like the movements in the Chinese martial art, tai chi, are the physical extensions of the spiritual goals of Zen Buddhism.

Of the many forms of yoga developed, two of the more popular in the West are Hatha, which emphasizes physical postures (*asanas*) and breathing-control techniques (*pranayama*), and Raja, which primarily involves meditation. A physical posture— say, the classic cross-legged, open-palmed "lotus" pose—is the embodiment of a mental state. In this case it is the position for meditation, enabling you to lengthen the spine and control deep breathing—that is, filling the lungs so that they can push down hard on the diaphragm. There are many positions, with names like cat, cobra, and tree, and all emphasize proper breathing. By controlling breath, you regulate *prana*, the Indian equivalent of the Chinese concept of *chi*, the body's vital energy. As in Chinese traditional medicine, in yoga to be healthy your flow of *prana* should be balanced.

I was once called to the ICU to see a youthful-appearing fifty-year-old with advanced coronary disease who was experiencing severe angina. He was quite upset and said that he had been a vegetarian for years and was an avid yoga practitioner who taught classes quite frequently. Yet here he was.

I probed further and found that all the male members of his family had had severe coronary problems, with many dying by the age of forty. Heart disease was simply his genetic lot in life. But because of his lifestyle and yoga practices, he could be considered as a candidate for reparative surgery only, rather than a heart transplant. And indeed, my yogi did very well with his operation and went home, with his own heart, in five days. Odds are that he is in a yoga pose as you read this.

At our Complementary Care Center, we use a modified yoga routine designed to prevent injury to the sternum area. Our therapists teach my open-heart surgery patients special positions and techniques for people with tender wounds and limited chest mobility. As with all our complementary medicine treatments, we have been conducting ongoing, long-term studies of the effects of yoga on these patients. So far group questionnaires show positive results, although yoga's effects on the hard endpoints that we are observing, including infection, depression, and long-term recovery rates, are much more difficult to assess. One of my major goals, though, is to plant enough seeds of hope in patients to encourage them to maintain therapies such as yoga once they go home.

I've also implemented dietary therapy with my patients. While patients differ in what foods and dietary supplements they may need, I generally favor an aggressive low-fat approach to what they eat. For those with coronary-artery disease, for example, I recommend a mostly vegetarian diet, suggesting a switch to fish, low-fat cheeses, yogurt, and soy-based tofu for protein. The only allowable oils, I advise, are extra-virgin olive oil and one tablespoon of flaxseed oil daily. If a bland oil is required for baking, use cold-pressed canola oil. I also encourage them to stick to a high-fiber, complex-carbohydrate diet that includes plenty of vegetables, grains, fruit, beans, and other legumes.

Another heart-disease–reversal diet that has shown positive results is that recommended by Dr. Lance Gould, a widely respected cardiologist and researcher at the Herman Hospital's Houston Center for Cardiovascular Medicine. Among Dr. Gould's main recommendations, are the following:

• Reduce fat intake to less than ten percent, which means removing virtually all identifiable fat from their food. Many no-fat, no-cholesterol foods, such as salad dressings, butter substitutes (not margarine), mayonnaise, cheeses, and other protein sources, are widely available, making supply an easy matter.

• Make salads and vegetables—steamed, boiled, but never fried—a mainstay of the diet. Beans and other legumes are a good source of vegetable protein, but they have a relatively high caloric content and therefore should be eaten in moderation.

• Maintain a protein source of at least 50 to 70 grams daily. Dr. Gould suggests non-fat dairy products, turkey and chicken breast, soy burgers, protein supplements, fish, beans, and on occasion the leanest red meats, such as buffalo. The most desirable fish are salmon and deep-water species such as swordfish and tuna, but these must always be grilled, baked, sauteed in wine or other liquids without oil or butter.

• Eliminate sugar and starches as much as possible. This includes fruits and juices, bread, potatoes, rice, pasta, and cereals. The goal is to be on the lean side.

• Take daily doses of niacin, which is vitamin B^3 and one of the oldest, cheapest ways to lower blood fats (lipids). Niacin doses must start low—250 mg—and gradually increase to one gram three times a day after meals. Potential side effects include itching, flushing, and a rise in potentially harmful liver enzymes. Immediate-release, not slow-release, niacin has the lowest risk of effects on the liver.

Along with such a regimen, Dr. Gould insists his patients not smoke, exercise regularly and take multi-vitamins daily, plus any cholesterol-lowering drugs prescribed by their physicians.

Radical changes in diet, such as those favored by Drs. Ornish and Gould, can be as tough for patients as getting through a major operation. I find that psychologically the best time to begin such a major lifestyle change is right after surgery. In addition to the dieting change, I advise patients to take vitamin supplements. Depending on their monitored needs, I usually recommend multi-vitamin and mineral supplements containing selenium, folic acid, the B-complex group, zinc, and copper. I also suggest extra doses of vitamins E and C for most patients, and also encourage magnesium, calcium, and an antioxidant called coenzyme Q10.

Many books and articles by Ornish, John McDougall, Bernard Siegel, Andrew Weil, and other physician-authors provide abundant facts about heart-healthy diets. I divide the pills into high- and low-priority categories, and patients may move on to the second-line additions if they are happy with the pills they already take.

Certain patients turn out to have special needs for certain vitamins. For example, when I transplanted a donor heart into Dr. Herbert Hoffner, a sixty-two-year-old ophthalmologist, I never expected his route to wellness would be folic acid and vitamin B[6].

Herbert had his first MI when he was forty-three. Eleven years later he had a second attack, followed by a third two years after that. His doctors attempted to do an angioplasty, but he arrested several times during the procedure and had to be brought back repeatedly with paddle shocks. By the time I saw him, he'd been in a coma for two weeks and was in sore need of an LVAD pump to bridge him to a transplant. During his recovery and while he waited for a new heart, Herbert was too weak to walk most of the time. So he couldn't socialize much with the other patients.

Early in his hospital stay, I suggested he try various complementary therapies, which he did. He liked therapeutic massage treatments, but the practice he was most committed to was dietary. For nearly twenty years, since his first attack, he had followed an extremely low-fat, low-sodium diet. Obviously, this regime by itself did not prevent further clotting, though if he hadn't been so careful about what he ate, his attacks might have been fatal.

"Still, it's crazy," he told me. "I've watched my diet like a hawk, and here I am on my third heart attack, facing a transplant. But I have a brother who had a heart attack years ago who's never stopped eating red meat or even smoking—and he's just fine. All he ever does to take care of himself is pop vitamins . . ."

"Why," I asked, "would someone who would knowingly abuse themselves in every way take vitamins?"

"Almost everyone on my mother's side has had a coronary in their forties, so we knew we had bad genes. When my brother had his attack at age twenty-nine, the rascal knew he lacked the willpower to shape up, so he argued that maybe megavitamin therapy could buy him salvation. He guessed right."

This was an important clue. In a family with a strong history of premature coronary disease, we were obliged to search for genetic defects, but now I knew that one or more of these vitamins seemed to reverse or halt the process. Diet, exercise, and avoidance of cigarettes, which Dr. Hoffner had practiced, did not.

Right after the transplant I referred him to a cholesterol specialist, who did blood tests and found that Hoffner's level of homocysteine, a protein-breakdown product, was extremely high. That was bad news because at high levels homocysteine will damage the blood vessels, which the body then tries to patch up with cholesterol. Elevated homocysteine levels are found in about one-fifth of the patients with coronary-artery disease; and transplant patients with elevated levels, as a study at the Cleveland Clinic Foundation shows, run an especially high risk of continued heart disease and blood clotting in the vessels.

The antidote for high homocysteine, it turns out, is B-complex vitamins and folic acid, which allow normal metabolism of proteins and prevent the abnormal accumulation of this toxic material. Because of his megavitamin program, Hoffner's delinquent brother had some of the highest folic acid levels measured and had only borderline elevated homocysteine. Hoffner's brother had stumbled onto the perfect treatment for his condition and so, despite his less diligent eating habits, had managed to preserve his heart. Once we got Dr. Hoffner on a megavitamin plan that emphasized folic acid and the B vitamins, particularly vitamin B^6, his homocysteine levels dropped dramatically to normal, and his health greatly improved.

When patients take charge, sometimes surgery can be prevented altogether. By the time I met Dr. Lou Angioletti, a world-renowned eye surgeon, and his twenty-two-year-old daughter, Lacey, she had already been diagnosed with idiopathic cardiomyopathy, which means an enlarged, weakened heart with no identifiable cause. They came to me for a formal consultation and advice about which complementary medicine could be beneficial. This pro-active family wanted to know what role they could play in ensuring her recovery.

"Tell me about yourself," I said.

A surgeon's daughter, familiar with our jargon, Lacey had already seen a battery of doctors, from cardiologists to hemotologists. She knew the drill. "Where do I start?" she said. "Medical or personal stuff?"

"Try personal—I read your chart," I said, glancing at her dad, "and Lou filled me in. He says you're an athlete."

"Was," Lacey answered with a shrug.

"Hey," I said sympathetically, "consider it an injury time-out. You'll get back to it."

Lou interjected, "That's what I keep telling her."

Lacey then described her first three years at Syracuse University, where she rowed for the varsity women's crew team, ran track, and played field hockey and volleyball. Then just as she was starting the fall semester, she separated from her boyfriend. Her physical problems started first with a fever, then vomiting and retention of fluids. She grew weak and tired. "I could barely get out of bed," she said, adding that she had to drop out of school and return home. Finally, Lacey had trouble breathing, and that's when her father took her to a hospital ER.

Tests showed her heart was overly large, severely weakened, and not working with anywhere near its strength of a year before when she rowed and ran in top form. Several well-known athletes have developed this condition, which nowadays kills about one percent of Americans, especially men. Lacey spent four days in the hospital, during which two clots in her heart were dissolved. Then she began months of rest and recuperation at home, but she wasn't showing much improvement. That's when I met her and her father—long divorced from Lacey's mother—and suggested that complementary medicine might help.

"There's hypnosis, yoga, meditation," I began, "certain vitamins."

"Dr. Oz," Lacey said, "I'm doing it all now, including vitamins and eating all the right things."

I realized that like most good athletes, she was highly focused and goal-oriented. "All right," I said, "but remember something. It's not only what you put in your mouth that heals you, but also what you put into your head."

Months later, well on her way to a strong recovery, Lacey told me those words stuck with her as a sort of mantra. Getting better suddenly became more of a mental than a physical challenge. Besides her dedication to such stress-lowering techniques as self-hypnosis and yoga, Lacey—on the advice of her father and another doctor—began to take low doses of an experimental growth-hormone drug, plus a daily mega-dose of the antioxidant coenzyme Q10. That was the turning point. Her heart apparently started to repair itself: the muscle became stronger and more normal in size, and its function greatly improved. The last I heard, she had finished college, was running again, and had launched a modeling career. The lesson here was obvious. For Lacey Angioletti, what worked best came from two worlds of medicine—an allopathic drug from one and a set of mind-calming and focusing exercises from the other.

I can't overstate the importance of a patient's attitude toward his or her illness and the long road to recovery. Somewhere in the process, the patient must decide to act, and must make a choice to participate in getting well. The mind must help the body.

Another complementary healing approach, homeopathy, actually puts the body in charge of healing itself. Its practitioners explain that by giving small amounts of substances or remedies—like quinine for malaria, or phosphate for nosebleeds—that cause symptoms similar to the ones the patient is experiencing, the body's self-healing mechanisms can overcome the original harmful problems. Whereas in conventional, allopathic medical practice, doctors, nurses, and others are trained to *fight* the symptoms of disease and illness, homeopaths work *with* the symptoms on the assumption that the symptoms are the body's way of fighting the disease.

Homeopathy began in Germany in the late eighteenth century when Samuel Hahnemann, a physician and chemist, started some experiments and treatment trials that were based on the doctrine of "like cures like." He became convinced that by using small doses of medicinal preparations mimicking symptoms of certain illnesses, he could produce in the patient a natural healing reaction. He also believed that the more subtle the medicine given, the higher its curative potency, which he likened to a spiritual, or vital, force. Held as a mutual belief by both doctor and patient, this approach to a cure may have helped harness the patient's own resources for healing. Hahnemann, who early in his career ran an asylum for the mentally ill, probably understood very well the importance of psychological factors in healing.

Patients are often surprised when I tell them that in America during the first half of the nineteenth century homeopathy was regarded as a highly effective treatment for many ailments. By successfully using algorithms to assess treatment outcomes, homeopathists actually gained a larger following than did conventional, orthodox medical practitioners, most of whom still relied on drugs, blistering, purging, and bleeding to fight illness.

Today, the homeopathic physician is trained to spot the one medicine, or group of complementary medicines—out of the collection of two thousand-odd substances in his well-tested pharmacopoeia—that the sick patient before him needs. However, there are two hallmarks of the homeopathist's approach to treatment: a recognition of small differences between one patient and another, and a belief that the human body be viewed as an integrated whole. Thus, homeopathy is "holistic," which contrasts with the analytical approach of orthodox medicine in examining and treating *parts* of the body, not the whole organism. Homeopathy's goal is to produce a balance in the biochemical workings of the entire body, or, as traditional medicine practitioners of the East would say, to encourage the body's vital forces to be in harmony.

All the therapies described in this book, used as adjuncts to conventional medicine, can broaden our power to heal and be healed. Many doctors are beginning to see the wisdom of addressing the whole patient—something complementary medicine can do in conjunction with conventional Western medicine—instead of just isolated symptoms, or as a body separated from a soul. By properly testing these therapies and strictly credentialing their practitioners, American hospitals might someday include both healing approaches in their menu of offerings.

🙞 10 🙜

Universal Healing

*"If one learns from others but does not think,
one will be bewildered.
If, on the other hand, one thinks but does not learn from others,
one will be in peril."*

—Confucius, *Analects* Book II

Recently, I visited China at the invitation of my father-in-law, Dr. Gerald Lemole, to help him do several demonstration open-heart surgeries. Beyond what I had read and seen in books, newspapers, movies, and documentaries, I had few preconceptions of what the country and culture were like. Nothing concrete and tangible, nothing I had seen firsthand—certainly not anything about the treatments they practiced in their traditional-medicine clinics.

The surgeries were performed without problems. We operated in a facility that was Western-oriented in its physical setup, and the Chinese doctors—all with solid allopathic training—seemed to be copying our methods and procedures quite well. Their instrumentation, however, though serviceable, was more rudimentary than ours. After the surgeries I asked our hosts if I could have a look at some of their traditional medical care. At first they were reluctant—perhaps they felt awkward or defensive about showing a foreigner their more ancient approaches to healing—but I finally won them over.

I was taken to a large medical center—a building several stories high—and escorted to a central screening area just past the entrance in the middle of the facility. I was told that half the building treated the more acute problems, like heart attacks or appendicitis, by using Western-based medicine and technology, while the other half treated patients with more chronic problems, like aching joints, colds, and headaches, with traditional Chinese medicine approaches. At the building's center, near the entrance, screeners were stationed to listen to patients and, based on their complaints, direct them either to the right or to the left. To me it was a very dramatic division of the two main ways humans treat illness. One was organ-based and pathology-oriented, developed to kill or counter disease in particular organs or parts of the body; and the other countered problems of pain and discomfort by trying to get the whole body back into healthy, energy-flowing balance again.

All Chinese practitioners, I was informed, regardless of which paradigm of medicine they ultimately followed, received the same first two years of training. They all studied physiology, anatomy, and all the other basic courses of any conventional medical school. By the end of that period of study, they could all speak the same technical language—both brain surgeons and acupressurists would understand such basic concepts as the location and function of organs or that carbohydrates produce energy quickly.

Then their approaches would diverge and might offer radically different interpretations of the same complaint. Someone might come in complaining of chest pains. Western medicine might diagnose the cause as heart disease, which could affect the liver and kidneys. Traditional medicine, on the other hand, might observe that the heart *chakra* is weak, creating insufficiencies that will result in imbalances in other *chakras*, leading to further dysfunction.

I once did open-heart surgery on an Armenian woman who was discharged without complications but came back complaining of having a very cold nose and overly warm feet. As a Western physician, how could I address those kinds of complaints? They didn't fit into any symptom complex I'm familiar with, so all I could tell her was that a lot of strange symptoms occur in patients after an open-heart operation. That's not much to offer a patient with a legitimate health complaint.

If I had easy access to traditional, or complementary, healers (as my Chinese counterparts do) I might hypothetically have been able to say, "Ah, cold nose and hot feet represent a classic deficiency in the third *chakra*," and then prescribe some herbs for the woman to take or recommend acupuncture. I could then, reverting to my Western research methods, study how effective the traditional treatment had been. If it worked well, I would not only know how to treat my next patient with this complaint, but I could also begin to ask patients if they had the same problem, so I could see if "third *chakra* deficiencies" were common after heart surgery.

That is exactly how I came to recognize and treat anorexia in open-heart surgery patients. I didn't really notice it much until my father-in-law let me in on a little secret of his. He had noticed that some of his patients were not hungry after surgery and suspected that the reason was because they had lost their sense of *taste*. By treating them with zinc, he was able to restore their taste sense and improve their appetites. Then I started asking patients if they had the problem, and many more than I expected did. Now questions about patients' sense of taste have become a routine part of my exam.

In the Chinese clinic I visited—one that's typical of thousands treating many millions of people in a country of more than a billion—I watched practitioners examine tongues and eyes, looking for clues to imbalance problems, then check pulses, and finally write out prescriptions for herbal and animal-based medicines. Other patients might be directed to an acupuncture practitioner. I followed one middle-aged man complaining of knee pain to an acupuncture room. The practitioner, a reed-thin older man, listened to the patient describe his symptoms, read the earlier diagnosis, then asked his subject to lie down on the treatment table. Needles and cupping were apparently called for. Cupping, which was once a common treatment in Europe, was done with heated glass cups placed over the skin around the knee, where they created a vacuum and literally sucked blood through the epidermis. Cupping, my translator told me, would increase blood flow and circulation in the knee and was particularly helpful for such conditions as rheumatism, lumbago, and stiff neck and shoulders.

Throughout the cupping procedure the patient appeared at ease. But I was then amazed by the aplomb with which he accepted the insertion of a dozen or so foot-long needles. Granted, acupuncture needles are so narrow that hardly a sting is felt when they puncture the skin, and the old healer had a practiced touch, a skill that takes many years to master. After jabbing a wire needle into a patient's skin, he would spin it back and forth at the other end with his thumb and forefinger. He appeared to be wiggling the wire, as if he were trying to catch something beneath the man's skin. Then snap! He'd catch it, let it go, and continue with the next needle. I was informed the "it" was some point of energy blockage in one of the body's meridians, or energy pathways. Before we left, I learned that this practitioner was reputed to be a master at relieving lower back pains by manipulating the needles on either side of the spine.

My next and last stop was at the clinic's herbal pharmacy, a large, busy room with rows of cabinets, each with many small drawers. These contained various herbs and dried parts of wild animals and insects. One drawer might contain one of many kinds of ginseng; another would hold bits of scorpion tail. There were hundreds, maybe thousands of different herbs, roots, flowers, pieces of tree bark, seeds, and natural oils. Attendants would take prescriptions, gather all ingredients ordered, then mix, crush, and beat them, and finally package the medicine. As I had seen in Thailand, Chinese patients seemed quite diligent in fol-

lowing instructions on how to prepare medications by boiling
and soaking the ingredients. In their cultures, taking responsibility for your own health is a much more time-consuming activity than it is in the West, where pill-popping is the medical
equivalent of fast food.

I came away from my visit to the clinic and to China impressed with their expeditious, two-system approach to health
care. As in the United States, most patients' complaints are
minor and chronic, so traditional healers can see, examine, and
dispatch many more patients at a cheaper cost than our science-
based, allopathic system makes possible. I don't see our developing the kind of mass-treatment approach to health care that I
saw in China, but it's likely we'll include the use of complementary practitioners once we find good ones that we trust. Then,
too, to have an efficient referral system between the two medical
systems we need to develop a common ground for understanding
each other—starting at the basic level of the vocabulary we use.
The Chinese have conveniently figured this out, since every
medical professional is steeped in the same knowledge during
the first two years of training.

My colleagues truly have their patients' best interests in
mind when they express concern that complementary therapies
are all hocus-pocus, that we're misleading patients. They say
there's no proof that these treatments work, so it's better not to
bother to try them. My argument is that if we're studying them
as scientists—as inquisitive investigators—then we'll find out
which kinds of complementary therapies work and which don't.
But we shouldn't have a double standard. If we applied the same
criteria to our system that we use to judge complementary medicine, our analytic process would paralyze us.

We make educated judgments about illnesses and treatments
all the time. We make "best guesses," and we ask for second and
third opinions. We often practice an inexact science because
there are still far too many unknowns and variables—and each
patient is a different organism with a different set of past and

present circumstances. It is because of these differences that computers cannot readily replace the human mind and touch of a doctor. And as doctors we could offer patients something extra by learning more about the world of complementary healing. We should consider it post-graduate medical study.

I believe that enough patients now want this dual system of care, so we in the medical establishment are going to have to deliver complementary treatments in a more formal way over the next decade. That's why we need the hard-science data, the rigorous clinical trials of these complementary therapies that we're attempting in our clinic. We're trying to bridge both worlds of medicine, the way I once dreamed many years ago in Istanbul of connecting two truths—from East and West—into some sort of common paradigm.

A Confucian saying I once heard draws a parallel between the truths of life and the blemishes in jade, since both provide an extra dash of beauty. That is, nothing is perfect, not even beauty. Similarly, modern medicine is not perfect, and may never be. Yet these gaps in our diagnostic skills, these imperfections or blemishes, if you will, affect our humanity, pushing us to find the best solutions for staying healthy and fighting disease and illness. I believe that as we move into the next century, we will view all medicine, old and new, as one universal healing endeavor, with blemishes from all quarters sometimes accepted. In such a spirit will we strive to perfect the many ways we heal ourselves.

EPILOGUE

This epilogue is an overview of the complementary medicine techniques that we are exploring at Columbia Presbyterian, along with some anecdotal and research data on how efficacious they might be. Since many of these therapies are only now, for the first time, being tested by Western scientific methods, it is too soon even to speculate on which ones will ultimately prove to be valuable healing tools, meriting a place in our conventional medical arsenal. I must also caution that since patients' needs and problems vary greatly, the regimens I describe here (including the nutritional, vitamin, chronic ailments, and mental health care recommendations) should never be adopted without the approval of a qualified physician.

The purpose of this epilogue, then, is not to prescribe or to promote alternative treatments but rather to offer patients whatever knowledge we have that can empower them to participate in their own care. A patient must become part of a team, working alongside the physician and other practitioners—from registered nurses to energy healers—to effect his or her own recovery.

A useful reference highlighting the patient's role in healing is Peggy Huddleston's *Prepare for Surgery, Heal Faster* (Angel River Press, 1996). An easy-to-read and useful summary of the evidence in support of and against many complementary therapies is Dr. Rosenfeld's *Guide to Alternative Medicine* (Fawcett Columbine, 1996). Specific centers that provide a comprehensive recovery program are listed at the end of this book and include programs led by Drs. Dean Ornish, Lance Gould, Herbert Benson, Andrew Weil, and Jon Kabat-Zinn. Also, my center welcomes telephone or E-mail requests for advice on who to see for particular ailments.

Columbia Presbyterian Complementary Medicine Services
Milstein 7-435, Columbia Presbyterian Medical Center
177 Fort Washington Avenue, New York, NY 10032
212 305-9628
mco2@columbia.edu

SPECIFIC THERAPIES

Music therapy

In our center, all patients are encouraged to listen via headphones to tapes playing the music of their choice or material we provide (Monroe Institute Binaural "Hemisync" Tapes, Faber, VA). Whichever option is selected, the patient begins listening to the tapes from the time of the first visit to the physician's office, and similar tapes are played during surgery. There is strong evidence that patients are subconsciously aware of what happens during surgery[1]; in our own clinic we've discovered that we can condition patients to respond one way or another depending on what we've played for them in the operating room. As a side benefit, the audiotapes also allow patients to block out the disturbing "illness" noises of the operating room and the intensive-care unit so they can stay focused on healing.

Hypnosis

Pre-operative hypnosis and meditation training can also help a patient feel more in control before, during, and after surgery. We did a study in which patients, selected blindly and randomly, were taught these techniques a few days before surgery.[2] The patients who learned and practiced them needed less pain medication than those who refused the treatment—and, indeed, some need *no* pain medication at all after leaving the intensive-care unit. Although the randomized trial showed no improvement in pain sensation overall, the hypnosis patients did report less anxiety.

All hospitals have psychiatry departments with staff members or psychologists trained in hypnosis, so you may want to ask for a referral. An informative book on this topic is written by Stanley Fisher, Ph.D., and is entitled *Discovering the Power of Self-Hypnosis* (Harper Collins, 1991).

Aromatherapy

Aromatherapy is one of the newer adjuncts to surgery, and one that many dismiss as somewhat frivolous. Yet the perfume industry has spent millions of dollars on scientific testing of smells and has amassed well-substantiated data showing that certain aromas, such as spicy ones, can make patients hypersensitive to pain, while others, such as flowery scents, dull the pain sensations. Already some American hospitals are using vanilla-scented oxygen in patients' nasal tubes, and more American medical centers are likely to join them as more of the European literature on this therapy appears in our medical journals. Aromatherapy can be hard to administer in a hospital setting but once home, many patients find it helpful in reducing stress and improving sleep.

Massage

Massage therapy is an area for more systematic study, though the anecdotal evidence of its effects are persuasive. Sixty percent of treated patients believe they have gained an independent positive effect from massage in our clinic, aside from feeling "good" during the session. Only two percent say they felt worse. In some hospitals massage is offered by staff practitioners, usually in half-hour or full-hour increments, and other hospitals will allow a massage therapist to visit an individual patient as an amenity. Even a nonprofessional massage by a family member can be helpful.

Reflexology, a technique concentrated on the feet and hands, attempts to affect internal organs by massaging the areas of the foot that correspond to as yet unmeasured "energy meridians." I am unaware of studies demonstrating the presence of these reflex relationships with the foot, but I do know that the density of nerve endings is higher in the extremities, making them especially sensitive to touch. I know of no risk from massage and have experimental evidence that lymphatic drainage is enhanced by rubbing the feet.

Yoga

My favorite therapy is yoga, since it allows meditation in conjunction with physical activity. Meditation alone is difficult for many Westerners, so focusing on the breathing and body first in order to center the mind can be much more effective. Better yet, virtually all patients, however ill, can perform some form of yoga, even if limited to deep breathing. Many yoga texts are available, but exercise tapes are easier to use and can be adapted readily to individual patients. I personally use the Brian Kest series.

Religion

We recognized early in our studies that more than fifty percent of patients think of religion as not just a spiritual guide, but also as a healing force. Our polls confirmed previous findings that ninety percent of hospitalized Americans are religious and would like to discuss the spiritual aspects of their care with their physicians. Few doctors offer this opportunity to patients voluntarily, but counseling can be arranged without much difficulty just by asking for a representative of the pastoral service.

Many religious leaders advocate love as a major healing force, and we try to highlight this message when we counsel critically ill patients. The most important study arguing for a positive therapeutic effect of intercessory prayer was conducted by Randolph Byrd in 1988. Almost four hundred intensive care unit patients were randomly chosen to receive either prayer or no prayer. The prayed-for patients had less need for respirators, antibiotics, and water pills. I have found Larry Dossey's writing particularly informative in this arena and am impressed by the anecdotal reports of patients. As no risk is apparent, I would make religion a part of my own therapy, especially if I were very ill.

Acupuncture

Acupuncture is rarely offered in hospitals outside the psychiatry wards, where its effects on substance abuse (and smoking) have been reasonably well documented in Western medical literature. But there is an intriguing litany of eyewitness reports of major operations being performed with only acupuncture for pain—inconceivable to most Western-trained physicians. A prominent cardiologist in our hospital, Isadore Rosenfeld, quite nicely describes an open-heart operation he witnessed in China without anesthesia—only acupuncture. Perhaps as Western experience of this ancient technique mounts, we will one day make it part of our own medical arsenal.

Although seemingly invasive, acupuncture by a licensed practitioner is an exceedingly safe intervention. I have recently collaborated with Dr. Soren Ballegaard, who has been sponsored by his government to evaluate the effectiveness of acupuncture in curbing angina pain. Because pain is a subjective phenomenon, assessment of efficacy is often difficult. However, Dr. Ballegard's preliminary data is encouraging enough that I believe patients who cannot undergo surgery or angioplasty for chest pain should be considered for this therapy.

EECP (enhanced external counterpulsation)

An alternative therapy for chronic angina that cannot be treated by any conventional means is enhanced external counterpulsation. Originating in China, EECP involves placing several blood-pressure cuffs on the lower extremities and sequentially constricting the legs to move blood to the heart. The patient is treated for several weeks prior to assessing the benefits. A cardiologist at my facility, Rohit Arora, studied 139 patients and found that, compared to the control group, those receiving EECP had a statistically significant improvement in exercise capacity without angina and an increase in ability to push the heart until ischemia (inadequate blood supply) occurs. I now encourage patients who cannot undergo more conventional treatments for angina such as ballooning (angioplasty) or surgery, to try EECP.

Chelation

I have seen patients suffering from severe angina reduce the pain to a tolerable level with chelation treatments. Yet virtually all eventually needed surgery. For some the chelation got too expensive or the hours receiving this "blood-cleansing" therapy became too boring for some or the effects diminished over time. Regardless, the lack of strong enough evidence supporting chelation therapy forces me to dissuade patients from seeking this therapy if more conventional treatments are available. For patients who cannot be managed by currently available methods, the rationale behind chelation is appealing. Since the side-effects appear marginal, I recommend these patients seek either EECP, acupuncture, or chelation. If the latter choice is made, they should contact the American Board of Chelation Therapy in Chicago for referrals to experienced practitioners in their region.

Energy (Therapeutic Touch)

The effects of acupuncture and homeopathy are theoretically based on energy meridians in the body. Some practitioners believe they can directly affect these energy states by the laying on of hands. Nurses in this country are often trained in this technique and anecdotally report favorable results. However, controlled studies in a clinical setting are very difficult to accomplish because the effects of therapeutic touch are hard to quantify.

In animal and plant tests, Bernard Grad has demonstrated some impact of an energy healer. And in our laboratories we have noticed interesting trends but have not identified a beneficial effect that we could reproduce. The Chinese *chi-gong* treatment has been reported to promote healing by affecting enzymatic relationships, but such an important observation requires much further study to give it credence. Clinically, several studies have shown some immunologic changes and accelerated healing of small wounds with therapeutic touch, but these alterations have not yet been correlated with accelerated recovery from illness. Since no side effects are known, I support all patients who have an inclination to pursue therapeutic touch, but I inform them of the unconvincing nature of the data to date.

Homeopathy

Homeopathy has long been practiced in this country, but has been pushed to the side by more conventional allopathic modalities. Its principle is the administration of exceedingly small doses of an active ingredient in a solvent for a "like-cures-like" effect. Instead of attacking the disease with the drugs of conventional medicine, homeopaths use substances—in the smallest doses possible—to stimulate the body to marshal its natural efforts to overcome disease.

This principle is very foreign to an allopathic physician like myself, but I have been lucky enough to see anecdotal beneficial results, which have raised my interest level. I would not dissuade a patient from pursing this avenue toward healing. However, since any ingested medicine that could help you could in theory hurt you as well, I strongly urge any patient interested in homeopathy to seek the guidance of a well-trained homeopath.

Nutritional recommendations

Since coronary-artery disease is this nation's major killer, I will describe dietary recommendations for this population. For many other ailments, especially cancer, diet provides the foundation for recovery and should be aggressively pursued. Authors like Michio Kushi (Avery Publishing) and Patrick Quillin (Nutrition Times Press) outline excellent programs, but any nutritional intervention should be supervised by an oncologist.

For atherosclerosis patients, no meat or dairy products are allowed except for skim milk and non-fat yogurt. The only oils allowed are extra-virgin olive oil and two tablespoons of flaxseed oil daily. These oils must be kept refrigerated and used within three months.

A complete-carbohydrate-based (starch) diet that includes vegetables, grains, legumes and beans, fruit, and soy products is advised. We emphasize that the patient should not just be removing foods from the diet, but also adding new staples that are high in fiber. The main course should move away from meat and poultry and toward beans, vegetables, and grains.

We have found that it is most effective to make dietary changes all at once—a paradigm shift that parallels the major operation the patient has just had. Before the dramatic effects on a patient's lifestyle have worn away, we try to influence them to embrace a new way of life, so the change seems more like a gain than a loss of the old staples. We hope that not only will coronary-artery disease risk be reduced but also that the patients will feel better overall.

Vitamin supplementation is often needed, since many of the processed foods we take today are devoid of the required levels of vitamins. In a Harvard nurses study, vitamin E (400 IU/daily) administered over two years led to a 46 percent reduction in the incidence of CAD, or coronary artery disease.[3] Vitamin C enhances the effectiveness of vitamin E, strengthens the endothelial surface, lessens thromboembolic risk, and raises the beneficial HDL cholesterol.[4] If possible, vitamin C should be taken twice a day in divided doses.

Magnesium, calcium, and selenium all play a major role in maintaining heart health. Calcium, in addition to its beneficial effects with osteoporosis,[5] reduces hypertension,[6] and diminishes the absorption of fats in the intestinal tract[7]. Magnesium can prevent irregular heart rhythms[8] and dilate blood vessels to improve circulation.[9] Low levels of selenium have been associated with heart disease and an increased risk of heart attack. L-carnitine facilitates the conversion of fats into energy in the myocardium and has been shown in randomized trials to increase exercise ability in patients with angina.[10] Coenzyme Q10 has been well studied in heart failure and angina and probably works most potently as an antioxidant,[11] although it may also improve the efficacy of the electron-transport chain. Both coenzyme Q10 and L-carnitine have been successfully used to help

keep the heart muscle alive during the course of a coronary
artery bypass graft, or CABG.[12]

Although these micronutrients are most likely safe—and we
have evidence supporting their efficacy—the appropriate selec-
tion and dosage should be done in conjunction with a health-
care provider. We often suggest that our patients who are free of
renal and liver dysfunction and not on blood-thinning medications take the following regimen:

Vitamin A with mixed carotenes	25,000 units/daily
Vitamin C	1,000 mg/daily
Vitamin E	400 IU/ daily
Coenzyme Q10	30 mg/3 times daily
L-carnitine	500 mg/2 times daily
Calcium citrate	1,000 mg/daily
Magnesium citrate	500 mg/daily
Folic acid	400 mcg/daily
EPA/DHA essential fatty acids	1gm/daily

Multivitamin containing selenium,
B-complex (including B[6] and B[12]),
zinc, and copper.

Although this is our basic program, individuals may have
specific abnormalities that mandate a more aggressive approach.
Since 21 percent of patients with coronary-artery disease have
high blood homocysteine levels,[13] all patients with coronary-
artery disease should have homocysteine levels checked and, if
they are elevated, be treated with folic acid (up to 5 mg/daily),
B[6] (up to 200 mg/daily), and sublingual B[12] (1,000 micrograms/
daily). Recently, one of my hospital administrators who had
undergone multiple angioplasties and failed an aggressive CAD-
reversal regimen, entered a Dean Ornish program, where his elevated homocysteine level was noted on screening and treated.
He has remained symptom-free for the past year.

In our center, diabetes is present in 30 percent of patients undergoing coronary artery disease. For these patients we recommend a

high-fiber, low-protein, complex-carbohydrate diet with chromium supplementation (200 microgram/daily). Chromium acts with insulin to aid the uptake of glucose into cells and may help treat the high glucose levels in diabetics.[14] Weight loss achieved through a complex-carbohydrate, high-fiber diet also has been effective in reducing insulin resistance in adult onset diabetes.[15]

Patients with elevated cholesterol that is resistant to dietary manipulation should use supplements to achieve a reduction. Niacin is the initial therapy recommended by the American Heart Association, although it often produces red-flushed skin. We start with the dose used in most studies (1,500 mg/daily). We avoid this by using inositol hexanicotinate. Then we add chromium, which not only lowers cholesterol but raises HDL and is especially effective when combined with niacin.[16] Gugulipid, an ayurvedic resin from the myrrh tree, has been found to lower cholesterol an average of 20 percent.[17] We recommend 25 mg of guggulsterone three times a day, although our experience on its effects is still anecdotal at this time. Then our patients embark on a second, more complex series of supplements only under the supervision of a physician.

The debate over estrogen supplements in post-menopausal women rages. Estrogens elevate HDL (the "good" cholesterol, small, dense particles that carry cholesterol in a stable form) and reduce LDL (the bad cholesterol, large, bulky, unstable forms that carry cholesterol). The major concern is the potential carcinogenic effects of estrogen, especially if unopposed by the usually present progesterone. Although estrogen alone can raise HDL, estrogen combined with progesterone can increase HDL levels significantly, while substantially lowering LDL levels. Another, less widely discussed effect of estrogen is its ability to modulate the contracting of coronary-artery vessels, which may be more important than the actual atherosclerosis in causing symptomatic coronary-artery disease.

Studies have shown some increased cancer risk with estrogen-replacement therapy. We may come to use naturally occurring forms of estrogen such as phytoestrogens to reduce coronary-artery disease in women. Whether or not to use hormone-replacement therapy—and what kind—is a decision that every woman should make individually, with the help of her doctor. Since many allopathic physicians are not up to date on the estrogen controversy, as a patient you should bring material on this topic to your physician to help with the discussion.

Specific Chronic Ailments and Their Treatments

Full restoration of health often eludes patients who have suffered a serious illness, and here complementary medicine may be especially helpful. Six chronic conditions that can reduce a patient's quality of life following an illness are poor wound healing, digestive complaints (including anorexia, constipation, and upset stomach), minor infections, musculoskeletal complaints, circulatory abnormalities, and such mental health complaints as stress and depression.

Wound healing

After surgical procedures, a superficial layer of cells will cover the wound and maintain sterility in the first twenty-four hours, although most surgeons prohibit active wetting of the wound for the first week. Native resistance to infection and proper nutrition will greatly facilitate healing. When a patient is malnourished (especially common in the elderly), wound healing is inhibited.[18] Diabetes can also slow the healing process, and desired treatment should include weight loss, using a high-complex carbohydrate, low-fat diet. High-fat diets will inhibit immune cell movement, thus predisposing the patients to systemic infections and poor wound healing.[19] Chromium supplements (200 mcg/daily) have also been argued to be beneficial, as well as vitamin C (1,000 mg/daily) and zinc (50 mg/daily).[20, 21, 22, 23] I do not recommend salves and I avoid putting anything in a wound which I would not put in an eye.[24]

Digestion

Many patients have a poor appetite following surgery, which can promote malnutrition. For many of these patients, the anorexia is associated with lack of smell and taste and can sometimes be treated with zinc (30 mg), vitamin A (10,000 IU, at least half of which should be mixed carotenes), and vitamin B complex (50 mg). A simple remedy for the upset stomach that sometimes occurs and can be responsible for anorexia is chamomile tea. Even if the patient is being treated for gastric hypoacidity, medications may be malabsorbed unless they are administered together with such substances as apple sauce, which slow their transit.

I encourage patients recovering from surgery to eat a high-fiber diet (30 gm/daily), although this can initially cause bloating with gas. The fiber diet can include oat bran or wheat bran cereal, which can be supplemented by psyllium (Metamucil) in fruit juice, in a dose that slowly increases from a half teaspoon to 2 teaspoons a day. Eating prunes and drinking 6 glasses of water daily will help reduce constipation. In general, constipation should not be treated with laxatives, which are a colonic irritant and from which the patient must be slowly weaned.

If these maneuvers fail, we have used with some success a mixture of the following items in the form of a drink:

    1 cup juice (orange, grapefruit)
    1 portion whole fruit (banana, peach, strawberries)
    1 tbsp flaxseed oil (refrigerated)
    1 tsp unprocessed wheat bran
    1 tsp psillium husks
    1/4 tsp vitamin C crystals

Infections

Many seriously ill patients develop chronic ailments, such as urinary-tract or minor respiratory-tract infections, that become chronic nuisances. When caused by viruses, these ailments are often not responsive to modern antimicrobial therapies. We recommend that these patients receive high doses of vitamin C (3–6 gm/daily),[25] echinacea,[26,27] licorice,[28] coenzyme Q10 [90–180 mg), and zinc (30 mg)[29] to allow the healing of inflamed tissue. These treatments are aimed at enhancing the body's natural immune function and should be carried out in addition to the more traditionally prescribed antimicrobials.

Musculoskeletal

Chronic aches and pains can be managed with some success using complementary techniques. As a first-time therapy, we recommend that our patients take calcium and magnesium. For those with chronically sore joints, we suggest a home remedy of 1 tbsp of cod liver oil, shaken vigorously in orange juice, then consumed every morning 30 to 60 minutes before breakfast. A final remedy with some support is the use of glucosamine sulfate 500 mg three times a day, which in theory will help to restore the naturally occurring gel that coats our joints and allows these biologic shock absorbers to function.[30,31]

Many patients gain relief by massaging arniflora gel into the site of soreness, as the arniflora serves as a topical anesthetic and an anti-inflammatory agent. The massage itself has therapeutic potential by improving lymphatic drainage[32] and relaxing muscle spasms. Patients who are minimally active lack the muscle stimulation that promotes proper lymphatic drainage and may benefit from reflexology (foot and hand) and massage (Swedish, Rolfing, and shiatsu). Some hospitals now offer massage combined with aromatherapy after surgery, and I strongly encourage patients to continue these therapies at home.[33] Simply being touched by another human being may have secondary, unquantifiable benefits.

Circulation

Circulatory problems are endemic in post-surgical patients. For clotting-related concerns, including phlebitis, we recommend vitamin E, which is a potent antioxidant as well as an anticoagulant. Foods rich in omega-3 fatty acids (cold-water fatty fish such as salmon, cod, herring, and mackerel) can reduce prostaglandins and are also anticoagulants.

Equally important is adequate activity. For elderly or feeble patients, yoga may be the ideal solution, since many simple poses require very little physical prowess and the deep breathing alone may be beneficial. Many yoga tapes and videos are commercially available, but as a start the patient can practice taking deep breaths in and out while attempting (with assistance) to touch the toes either in bed or while standing. Another technique being used with anecdotal success is "assisted bouncing," in which a patient sits on a trampoline and is gently and carefully pushed up and down.

Herbal circulatory aids are often recommended, including ginkgo biloba (40–60 mg three times a day),[34] which may also improve hearing, pycnogenol (50 mg twice a day of grape seed extract),[35] cayenne (1 capsule per meal), and lecithin, a prostaglandin inhibitor that reduces inflammation and increases cholesterol excretion.

Patients with heart disease often need diuretic therapy, which I prefer to begin with such gentle natural diuretics as parsley and vitamin C. With all diuretics, increased intake of dried fruits, peanuts, potatoes, spinach, or pumpkin seeds should be encouraged to maintain adequate potassium intake. For patients in heart failure, coenzyme Q10 has been carefully studied[36] and may improve cardiac function in this difficult-to-evaluate population. I recommend that patients take 60-to-120 mg with each meal; however, this compound can have erratic intestinal absorption. L-carnitine (750–1,000 mg twice a day) is another popular remedy which has been well studied in claudication (peripheral vascular disease)[37] and in congestive heart failure.[38]

Mental illness

Some of the most debilitating problems in post-surgical patients are mental. Lethargy can be managed with L-tyrosine, which increases norepinephrine levels,[39] and by the replacement of traditional caffeinated teas with green teas, which are also antioxidants. Memory problems, which are also part of this symptom complex, can be treated with phosphatidyl choline,[40] zinc (30 mg/daily), and ginko biloba (40–60 mg three times a day).[41]

In some people depression can be treated successfully with St. John's wort (4:1 hypericum, 300 mg three times a day). One study tested 105 depressed patients randomly assigned to receive either St. John's wort or a placebo. In the St. John's wort group, depression was reduced 55 percent versus 29 percent in the control group over a four-week treatment period.[42] Caffeinated beverages can promote depression, especially in amounts greater than four cups of coffee a day.[43] Vitamins—folic acid (800 mcg), B[12] (1,000 mg/daily), selenium (100 mcg/daily),[44] B-complex (50 mg) and magnesium (500 mg)—may help lift a patient's mood. Moreover, the headaches the patients often suffer can be treated with the herb feverfew.[45]

For insomnia, valerium,[46] 5-hydroxytryptophan (5 HTP), [47] and melatonin have been advocated and may have less side effects than prescription medications. The stress that often causes insomnia can be managed by yoga and audiotapes, which are often used for patients undergoing major surgical procedures to provide a calming environment. The anxiety that often accompanies insomnia can be reduced with glutamine and thiamine, the latter of which should be taken in the morning to avoid overly vivid dreams.

NOTES

1. Bennett HL. The mind during surgery: the uncertain effects of anesthesia. *Advances* 9:5–16, 1993.

2. Ashton RA, Whitworth GC, Seldomrige JA, Shapiro PS, Michler RE, Smith CR, Rose EA, Fisher S, Oz MC. Self-hypnosis reduces anxiety following coronary artery bypass surgery: a prospective, randomized trial. *J Cardiovascular Surgery* 1997;38:69–75.

3. Stampfer MJ. Vitamin E consumption and the risk of coronary disease in women. *NEJM* 328:1444–49, 1993.

4. Rath M, Pauling L. Hypothesis: Lipoprotein(a) is a surrogate for ascorbate. *Proc Nat Aced Sciences* 87(16):6204–6207, 1990.

5. Chapuy MC, Vitamin D^3 and calcium to prevent hip fractures in elderly women. *NEJM* 327:1637–42, 1992.

6. Hatton DC. Dietary calcium and blood pressure in experimental models of hypertension. *Hypertension* 23:513–30, 1994.

7. Garland C. Dietary vitamin D and calcium and risk of colorectoral cancer. *Lancet* 2:307–9, 1985.

8. England MR, Gordaon G, Salem M, Chernow B. Magnesium administration and dysrythmias after cardiac surgery. A placebo-controlled, double-blind, randomized trail. *JAMA* 268:2395–2402, 1992.

9. Seelig MS, Heggtveit HA. Magnesium interrelationships in ischemic heart disease. *Am J Clin Nutrition* 27(1):59–79, 1974.

10. Cherichi A. Effects of L-carnitine on exercise tolerance in chronic, stable angina: A multicenter, double-blind, randomized, placebo controlled crossover study. *Int J Clin Pharmocol Ther Toxicol* 23 (10): 569–72, 1985.

11. Hanaki Y, Sugiyama S, Ozawa T. Ratio of LDL lipoprotein cholesterol to ubiquinone as a coronary risk factor. *NEJM.* 325(11):814–815, 1991.

12. Silverman NA, Schmitt G, Vishwanath M.: Effect of carnitine on myocardial function and metabolism following global ischemicia. *Ann Thorac Surg* 40:20–25, 1985.

13. Boers GHJ. Hyperhomocysteinemia: A newly recognized risk factor for vascular disease. *Netherlands J Med* 45:34–41, 1994.

14. Anderson RA. Chromium, glucose intolerance, and diabetes. *Biol Trace Elem Res.* 32:19–24, 1992.

15. Anderson JW, Ward K. High-carbohydrate, high fiber diets for insulin-treated men with diabetes mellitus. *Am J Chin Nutr* 32:2312–21, 1979.

16. Urberg M, Benyi J, John R. Hypercholesterolemic effects on nicotinic acid and chromium supplementation. *J Fam Practice* 27(6): 603–6, 1988.

17. Nityanand S, Sriastava JS, Asthana OP. Clinical trials with gugalipid: a new hypolipidaemic agent. *J Assoc Phys India* 37:321–9, 1989.

18. Morely JE. *Am J Med.* 81:670, 1986.

19. RS Sparkman, Ed. The healing of surgical wounds: State of the art in the ninth decade of the 20th century. American Cyanamid Co., 1985: 75–80, 119.

20. Taylor TV. Ascorbic acid supplementation in the treatment of pressure sores. *Lancet* 1974; 2:544–46.

21. Seifter E. Impaired wound healing in streptozotocin diabetes. Prevention by supplemental vitamin. *Ann Surg* 1981; 194:42–50.

22. Goldstein R. Effect of vitamin E and allopurinol on lipid peroxide and glutathione level in acute skin grafts. *J Inves Dermatol* 1990; 95:470–5.

23. Hallbook T, Hedelin H. Zinc metabolism and surgical trauma *Br J Surg* 1977;64:271–73

24. Archer HG. A controlled model of moist wound healing: comparison between semi-permeable film, antiseptics, and sugar paste. *J Exp Pathol* 1990;71:155–70.

25. Scott J. On the biochemical similarities of ascorbic acid and interferon. *J Theor Biol* 1982;98:235–8.

26. Mose J. Effect of echinacin on phagocytosis and natural killer cells. *Med Welt.* 1983;34:463–7.

27. Wacher A, Hilbig W. Virus inhibition by echinacea purpurea. *Planta Medica* 1978; 33:89–102.

28. Armanini D. Further studies on the mechanism of the mineralocorto-coid action of licorice in humans. *J Endocrinol Invest* 1996;19:624–9.

29. Gershwin M, Beach R, Hurley L. Trace metals, aging, and immunity. *J Am Ger Soc.* 1983;31:374–8.

30. Mueller-Fabender H. Glucosamine sulfate compared to ibuprofen in osteoarthritis of the knee. *Osteoarthritis and Cartilage* 1994;2:61–69.

31. Reichelt A, Forster KK, Fischer M, et al. Efficacy and safety of intra-musuclar Glucosamine Sulfate in osteoarthritis of the knee. *Drug Research* 1994;44 (1):75–80.

32. Brace RA, Taylor AE, Guyton AC. Time course of lymph protein con-centration in the dog. *Microvascular research* 1997;14:243–249.

33. Oz MC, Lemole EJ, Oz LJ, Whitworth GC, Lemole GM. Treating coronary artery disease with cardiac surgery and complementary therapy. *Medscape Women's Health* (http://www.medscape.com/1(10), 1996.

34. Kleijnen J. Ginkgo biloba. *Lancet* 1992;340:1136 39.

35. Rong Y. Pycnogenol protects vascular endothelial cells from t-butyl hydroperoxide induced oxidant injury. *Biotechnol Ther* 1994;5:117–26.

36. Langsjoen PH, Vadhanavikit S, Folkers K. Response of patients in classes III and IV of cardiomyopathy to therapy in a bind and crossover trial with coenzyme Q10. *Proc Natl Acad Sci* 1985;82:4240–4244.

37. Brevetti G. Increases in walking distance in patients with peripheral vascular disease treated with L-carnitine: A double blind, cross-over study. *Circulation* 1988;77:767–773.

38. Cherchi A. Effects of L-carnitine on exercise tolerance in chronic stable angina. *Int J Clin Pharmacol Ther Toxicol* 1985;23:569–72.

39. Gibson C, Gelenberg A. Tyrosine for depression. *Adv Biol Psychiat* 1983; 10:148–59.

40. Cohen BM. Decreased brain choline uptake in older adults; an in vivo proton magnetic resonance spectroscopy study. *JAMA* 1995;274(11): 902–907.

41. Hoyer S. Possibilities and limits of therapy of cognition disorders in the elderly. *Z Gerontol Geriatr* 1995;28:457–62.

42. Harrer G, Sommer H. Treatment of mild/moderate depression with Hypericum. *Phytomedicine* 1994;1:3–8.

43. Kreitsch K. Prevalence, presenting symptoms, and psychological char-acteristics of individuals experiencing a diet-related mood disturbance. *Behav Ther* 1988;19:593–604.

44. Benton D. The impact of selenium supplementation on mood. *Biologi-cal Psychiatry* 1991;29:1092–98.

45. Murphy JJ. Randomized double blind placebo controlled trial of fever-few in migraine prevention. *Lancet* 1988; 2:189–92.

46. Lindahl O. Double blind study of a valerian preparation. *Pharmacol Biochem Behav* 1980; 32:1065–6.

47. Wyatt RJ, Zarcone V, Engleman K, Dement WC, Snyder F, Sjoerdsma A. Effects of 5-hydroxytryptophan on the sleep of normal human subjects. *Electroencephalography and Clinical Neurophysiology* 1971; 30: 505–9.

FURTHER READINGS

This is by no means a complete or exhaustive list of readings about various complementary medicine therapies and some of the issues and topics I discuss in *Healing from the Heart*. However, these books, magazines, and professional journals should prove helpful to patients and interested lay readers, as well as to medical practitioners and professionals in other related fields.

BOOKS

Achterberg, Jeanne, Barbara Dossey, and Leslie Kolkmeier. *Rituals of Healing: Using Imagery for Health and Wellness*. New York: Bantam Books, 1994.

Ackerman, Diane. *A Natural History of the Senses*. Avenel, N.J.: Random House Value Publishing, 1993.

Barnard, Neal. *Food for Life: How the New Four Food Groups Can Save Your Life*. New York: Crown Publishers, 1993.

Bassano, Mary. *Healing with Music and Color: A Beginner's Guide*. York Beach, Me.: Samuel Weiser, 1992.

Beinfield, Harriet. *Between Heaven and Earth: A Guide to Chinese Medicine*. New York: Ballantine Books, 1990.

Benson, Herbert. *The Relaxation Response*. New York: William Morrow, 1975.

Benson, Herbert, and Eileen M. Stuart. *The Wellness Book: The Comprehensive Guide to Maintaining Health and Treating Stress-Related Illness*. New York: Simon & Schuster, 1992.

Blevi, Viktor, and Gretchen Sween. *Aromatherapy*. New York: Avon Books, 1993.

Brennan, Barbara Ann. *Hands of Life: A Guide to Healing Through the Human Energy Field*. New York: Bantam Books, 1987.

Burton Goldberg Group. *Alternative Medicine: The Definitive Guide*. Puyallup, Wash.: Future Medicine Publishing, 1993.

Capra, Fritjof. *The Tao of Physics: An Exploration of the Parallels Between Modern Physics and Eastern Mysticism*. Boston: Shambhala, 1975.

Chopra, Deepak. *Perfect Health: The Complete Health Mind-Body Guide*. New York: Harmony Books, 1990.

Christiansen, Alice. *The American Yoga Association Beginner's Manual*. St. Louis: Fireside Books, 1987.

Crandall, Joanne. *Self-Transformation Through Music*. Wheaton, Ill.: Theosophical Publishing House, 1988.

Csikszentmihalyi, Mihaly. *Flow: The Psychology of Optimal Experience*. New York: HarperCollins, 1990.

Dossey, Larry. *Meaning & Medicine: Lessons from a Doctor's Tales of Breakthrough and Healing*. New York: Bantam Books, 1991.

Dossey, Larry. *Prayer Is Good Medicine: How to Reap the Healing Benefits of Prayer*. New York: HarperCollins, 1996.

Eisenberg, David, with Thomas Lee Wright. *Encounters with Qi: Exploring Chinese Medicine*. New York: W.W. Norton, 1995.

Epstein, Gerald. *Healing Visualizations: Creating Health with Imagery*. New York: Bantam Books, 1989.

Foster, Steven. *Herbal Renaissance: Growing, Using and Understanding Herbs in the Modern World*. Layton, Ut.: Smith, Gibbs, 1993.

Frawley, David. *Ayurvedic Healing: A Comprehensive Guide*. Sandy, Ut.: Passage Press, 1989.

Fritz, Sandy. *Mosby's Fundamentals of Therapeutic Massage*. St. Louis: Mosby-Year Book, 1995.

Gach, Michael Reed. *Acupressure's Potent Points: A Guide to Self-Care for Common Ailments*. New York: Bantam Books, 1990.

Gladstar, Rosemary. *Herbal Healing for Women*. New York: Simon & Schuster, 1993.

Golan, Ralph. *Optimum Wellness*. New York: Ballantine Books, 1995.

Hamilton, Kirk. *Clinical Pearls in Nutrition and Preventive Medicine*. Sacramento, Cal.: IT Services, 1997.

Kabat-Zinn, Jon. *Full Catastrophe Living: Using the Wisdom of Your Body and Mind to Face Stress, Pain, and Illness*. New York: Dell, 1991.

Kabat-Zinn, Jon. *Wherever You Go There You Are: Mindfulness Meditation in Everyday Life*. New York: Hyperion, 1994.

Lockie, Andrew. *The Family Guide to Homeopathy: Symptoms and Natural Solutions*. New York: Simon & Schuster, 1993.

Lundberg, Paul. *The Book of Shiatsu*. New York: Simon & Schuster, 1992.

McDougall, John. *The McDougall Program for a Healthy Heart: Life-Saving Approach to Preventing and Treating Heart Disease*. New York: Dutton, 1996.

McDougall, John, and Mary McDougall. *The New McDougall Cookbook*. New York: Dutton, 1993.

Mindell, Earl. *Earl Mindell's Good Food as Medicine*. New York: Simon & Schuster, 1994.

Moyers, Bill. *Healing and the Mind*. New York: Doubleday, 1993.

Norman, Laura. *Feet First: A Guide to Foot Reflexology*. New York: Simon & Schuster, 1988.

Ornish, Dean. *Dr. Dean Ornish's Program for Reversing Heart Disease*. New York: Ballantine Books, 1990.

Ornish, Dean. *Everyday Cooking with Dr. Dean Ornish: 150 Easy, Low-Fat, High-Flavor Recipes*. New York: HarperCollins, 1996.

Pizzorno, Joseph, and Michael Murray. *Encyclopedia of Natural Medicine*. Rocklin, Cal.: Prima Publishing, 1991.

Prevention Magazine Health Books. *New Choices in Natural Healing: Over 1,800 of the Best Self-Help Remedies from the World of Alternative Medicine*. Emmaus, Pa.: Rodale Press, 1995.

Reid, Daniel. *The Complete Book of Chinese Health and Healing*. Boston: Shambhala, 1994.

Sadler, Julie. *Aromatherapy*. New York: Sterling Publishing, 1994.

Shealy, C. Norman, consultant ed. *The Complete Family Guide to Alternative Medicine: An Illustrated Guide to Natural Healing*. Rockport, Me.: Element Books, 1996.

Siegel, Bernard. *Love, Medicine, and Miracles*. New York: Harper & Row, 1986.

Toussaint, Casserine. *Conquering Heart Disease: New Ways to Live Well Without Drugs or Surgery*. Boston: Little, Brown, 1994.

Ullman, Dana. *Discovering Homeopathy: Your Introduction to the Science and Art of Homeopathic Medicine*. Berkeley, Cal.: North Atlantic Books, 1991.

Weil, Andrew. *Eight Weeks to Optimum Health*. New York: Knopf, 1997.

Weil, Andrew. *Natural Health, Natural Medicine*. Boston: Houghton Mifflin, 1990.

Weiner, Michael, and Kathleen Goss. *The Complete Book of Homeopathy*. Garden City, N.Y.: Avery Publishing, 1989.

Werbach, Melvyn. *Healing Through Nutrition*. New York: Harper-Collins, 1993.

MAGAZINES AND JOURNALS

Advances: The Journal of Mind-Body Health
Alternative Health Practitioner
Alternative Therapies in Health and Medicine
Journal of Alternative and Complementary Medicine
Natural Health
New Age Journal
Total Health

NEWSLETTERS

Dr. Stephen Sinatra's *HeartSense*
Phillips Publishing, Inc.
P.O. Box 60042
7811 Montrose Rd.
Potomac, MD 20859
800-211-7643

Dr. Andrew Weil's *Self Healing*
Thorn Communications
42 Pleasant St.
Watertown, MA 02172
612-926-0200

Dr. Julian Whitaker's
Health and Healing
Phillips Publishing, Inc.
P.O. Box 60042
7811 Montrose Rd.
Potomac, MD 20859
800-539-8219

Dr. Jonathan Wright's *Nutrition and Healing*
Publishers Mgt. Corp.
P.O. Box 84909
Phoenix, AZ 85071
800-526-0559 or 602-252-4477

RESOURCES

Academy for Guided Imagery
Box 2070
Mill Valley, CA 94942
800-726-2070
Web site: www.healthy.net/agi

American Academy of
    Medical Acupuncture
5820 Wilshire Blvd., Suite 500
Los Angeles, CA 90036
800-521-2262

American Association of
    Naturopathic Physicians
2366 Eastlake Ave., E., Suite 322
Seattle, WA 98102
206-323-7610

American Chiropractic Association
1701 Clarendon Blvd.
Arlington, VA 22209
800-986-4636
Web site: www.amerchiro.org/aca

American Holistic
    Medical Association
4101 Lake Boone Trail,
    Suite 201
Raleigh, NC 27607
919-787-5181

American Massage Therapy
    Association
820 Davis St., Suite 100
Evanston, IL 60201-4444
847-864-0123

American Yoga Association
513 S. Orange Ave.
Sarasota, FL 34236
800-226-5859

Ayurvedic Institute
11311 Menaul NE, Suite A
Albuquerque, NM 87112
505-291-9698

Bastyr University
14500 Juanita Drive NE
Bothwell, WA 98011
206-523-9505

Born Preventative Health Care
    Clinic
2687 44th Street, SE
Grand Rapids, MI 49512
616-455-3550

Center for Mind-Body Medicine
Dr. James Gordon, Director
5225 Connecticut Ave., NW,
    Suite 414
Washington, DC 20015
202-966-7338

Community and Family
    Medicine
Barrie Cassileth, Consulting
    Professor
Duke University Medical Center
Chapel Hill, NC 27514
919-942-8500

Complementary Care Center
Dr. Mehmet Oz and Jery
    Whitworth, Co-directors
Columbia Presbyterian
    Medical Center
Milstein Hospital Bldg.
177 Fort Washington Ave.
New York, NY 10032
212-305-9628

Elisabeth Kubler-Ross Center
SRA, Box 28
Head Waters, VA 24442
703-396-3441

Fetzer Institute, Inc.
9292 West KL Ave.
Kalamazoo, MI 49009
616-375-2000

Herb Research Foundation
1007 Pearl St., Suite 200
Boulder, CO 80302
800-748-2617

International Association of Yoga
    Therapists
109 Hillside Ave.
Mill Valley, CA 94941
415-381-0876

International Foundation for
    Homeopathy
2366 Eastlake Ave., E, Suite 325
Seattle, WA 98102
425-776-4147

International Institute of
    Reflexology
P.O. Box 12642
St. Petersburg, FL 33733
813-343-4811

Mind/Body Medical Institute
Deaconess Hospital
1 Deaconess Rd.
Boston, MA 02215
617-632-9525

National Center for Homeopathy
801 N. Fairfax St., Suite 306
Alexandria, VA 22314
703-548-7790
Web site: www.healthy.net/nch

Office of Alternative Medicine,
  National Institutes of Health
900 Rockville Pike
Bldg. 31, Rm. 5-B-38
Bethesda, MD 20892
800-531-1794

Oncara Intercultural Center
P.O. Box 70
Brandon, VT 05733
802-388-1237

Pacific Institute of Aromatherapy
Box 6723
San Rafael, CA 94903
415-479-9121

People's Medical Society
462 Walnut St.
Allentown, PA 18102
800-624-8773

Preventive Medicine
  Research Institute
Dr. Dean Ornish, Director
900 Bridgeway, Suite 2
Sausalito, CA 94965
415-332-2525, ext. 222

Pritikin Longevity Center
2811 Wilshire Blvd., Suite 410
Santa Monica, CA 90402
800-421-9911

Program for Preventing or
  Reversing Coronary
  Heart Disease
Dr. K. Lance Gould,
  Professor of Medicine
University of Texas
  Medical School
6431 Fannin, Room 4.258 MSB
Houston, TX 77030
713-500-6611

Reflexology Research
P.O. Box 35820
Albuquerque, NM 87176
800-624-8773

Shealy Institute for
  Comprehensive Health Care
1328 E. Evergreen St.
Springfield, MO 65803
417-865-5940

St. Helena Hospital &
  Health Center
P.O. Box 250
Deer Park, CA 94576
800-358-9195

University of Maryland
  Pain Center
Dr. Brian Berman, Director
University of Maryland School of
  Medicine
Baltimore, MD 21201
410-706-3100

Whitaker Wellness Institute, Inc.
4321 Birch St.
Newport Beach, CA 92660
714-851-1550

ACKNOWLEDGMENTS

This work arose from life experiences that would not have been as informative or enjoyable without the guidance and help of in numerable friends. This list is an attempt to thank several groups of colleagues. In no way is the list complete, although we have tried to list as many individuals as possible. We are most indebted to countless patients who shared their lives with us and have allowed us to document their battles with life-threatening illnesses. We hope our forays into complementary medicine enable these challenges to result in personal growth rather than only memories of overcome obstacles. Many of you are listed by name in the text, and we hope to maintain friendships with the many whom we could not include but whose stories nevertheless deserve to be told.

Lisa and my family, especially our parents Mustafa and Suna Oz and Gerald and Emily Jane Lemole, have provided the guidance that laid the seeds from which our search grew. We have enjoyed lifelong support and friendship from our siblings, Seval, Nazlim, Laura, Emily, Michael, Samantha, and Christopher.

Thanks to our young children, Daphne, Arabella, and Zoe, for sacrificing the time with us needed to create the book.

My professional colleagues, who have almost all become personal friends as well, have sacrificed to teach me the essentials of surgical practice and to infuse in a young and inquisitive man the "chi" of a surgeon. I was blessed to be mentored by Dr. Eric Rose, who demonstrated patience and guidance both within and outside the operating theater. Drs. Craig Smith, Jan Quaegebeur, and Henry Spotnitz teamed up to complete my cardiac surgical education. Drs. Ken Steinglass and Mark Ginsberg taught me my father's specialty. Drs. Roman Nowygrod, David Stern, and David Pinsky were tireless teachers, especially in my early years as a surgical investigator. Dr. Bashir Zikria, a brave and brilliant scientist, surgeon, and religious leader, provided insights that stimulated me to seek new adventures in our field.

The complementary medicine team, without which the systematic management of patients desiring complementary medicine would not have been feasible, deserves credit for the program's rapid growth. In particular, Jery Whitworth, with whom I have grown tremendously, provided the organization and the life energy to keep the center on track. Sarah Shaines, Geri Messer, and Gil Binenbaum helped coordinate the growth together with the help of many practitioners to whom I and many of my satisfied patients are eternally grateful. Volunteers like Julie Motz, medical students, and aspiring physicians selflessly dedicated countless hours to our research efforts. Drs. Dean Ornish and Sandy McClannahan were pioneers in the field to whom I owe a tremendous intellectual debt, especially for awakening me to the joys of yoga.

My coaches on athletic fields, where many of my formative battles were waged, include Steve Hyde, Harry Baetjer, John Pearson, and George Stetson. My spiritual guides included Prescott Rogers, Hakki Oz, Cezmi Mutlu, and Ivan Kronenfeld. I am especially indebted to Ivan and Anne for helping conceive the idea for the book and for guidance during my navigation of the sometimes turbulent complementary medicine waters.

Complementary medicine cannot work without the cooperation of the entire patient-care team. This includes my anesthesiologist colleagues, the operating room nurses led by Flora Wong, the intensive care nurses, and the floor nurses. The physician's assistants and residents played a large role in the clinical success of the many patients enrolled in our program. In particular, the office staff, especially Lidia Nieves, Diane Amato, Peggy Haubert, and Craig Evans has provided a broad base of support.

The LVAD crew, including Kathy Catanese, Margaret Flannery, Mike Gardocki, Howard Levin, Asim Choudhri, and Donna Mancini, whose teamwork I cherish so deeply, was open-minded enough to allow critically ill patients to try complementary medicine. The transplant community, including physicians, nurse coordinators, social workers, and patients, have provided grassroots support for complementary medicine, especially in its early years at Columbia Presbyterian. Their support was reinforced by the guidance of the Presbyterian Hospital and Columbia University administrations, who have agreed to study the modalities in question in a scientifically sound fashion before passing judgment. Many of the early debates leading to this decision originated in the complementary medicine screening committee, which included Drs. Don Kornfeld and Michael Leahey.

My friends in the press, who carefully and eloquently described our efforts, made much of our growth possible. Chip Brown, whose magical article in the *New York Times Magazine* captured the essence of the program, and Steven Dubner have remained close friends. The public relations offices of the university and especially the hospital have worked overtime to make our program accessible to interested parties. Michaela Hamilton, Elisa Petrini, Mitch Douglas, and Reid Boates have provided the guidance through the literary world needed to create a finished work.

Finally, my co-authors, Lisa and Ron, kept the light burning during the dark days of this manuscript's creation. Ron, a tireless and gifted writer, has an inner knowledge of complementary medicine and was the perfect partner for a demanding heart surgeon. My partner in life, Lisa, has been the bedrock on which the LVAD and complementary medicine centers were built. She has been at my side during my most painful ordeals with sick patients and has always resuscitated me to rejoin the battle. Thank you.

INDEX